Polypharmacy

Guest Editor

HOLLY M. HOLMES, MD

CLINICS IN GERIATRIC MEDICINE

www.geriatric.theclinics.com

May 2012 • Volume 28 • Number 2

SAUNDERS an imprint of ELSEVIER, Inc.

W.B. SAUNDERS COMPANY
A Division of Elsevier Inc.

1600 John F. Kennedy Blvd., Suite 1800. Philadelphia, Pennsylvania 19103-2899

http://www.theclinics.com

CLINICS IN GERIATRIC MEDICINE Volume 28, Number 2
May 2012 ISSN 0749–0690, ISBN-13: 978-1-4557-3868-7

Editor: Yonah Korngold

Clinics in Geriatric Medicine (ISSN 0749-0690) is published quarterly by Elsevier Inc., 360 Park Avenue South, New York, NY 10010-1710. Months of issue are February, May, August, and November. Business and Editorial Offices: 1600 John F. Kennedy Blvd., Suite 1800, Philadelphia, PA 191023-2899. Periodicals postage paid at New York, NY, and additional mailing offices. Subscription prices is $257.00 per year (US individuals), $448.00 per year (US institutions), $131.00 per year (US student/resident), $334.00 per year (Canadian individuals), $559.00 per year (Canadian institutions), $355.00 per year (foreign individuals) and $559.00 per year (foreign institutions). Foreign air speed delivery is included in all *Clinics* subscription prices. All prices are subject to change without notice. POSTMASTER: Send address changes to *Clinics in Geriatric Medicine,* Elsevier Health Sciences Division, Subscription Customer Service, 3251 Riverport Lane, Maryland Heights, MO 63043. Telephone: 1-800-654-2452 (U.S. and Canada); 314-447-8871 (outside U.S. and Canada). Fax: 314-447-8029. E-mail: journalscustomerservice-usa@elsevier.com (for print support) or journalsonlinesupport-usa@elsevier.com (for online support).

Reprints. For copies of 100 or more, of articles in this publication, please contact the Commercial Reprints Department, Elsevier Inc., 360 Park Avenue South, New York, New York 10010-1710. Tel.: (212) 633-3812; Fax: (212) 462-1935, email: reprints@elsevier.com.

Clinics in Geriatric Medicine is covered in *MEDLINE/PubMed (Index Medicus), EMBASE/Excerpta Medica, Current Contents/Clinical Medicine (CC/CM)*, and the *Cumulative Index to Nursing & Allied Health Literature.*

Printed in the United States of America

Transferred to Digital Printing, 2012

Contributors

GUEST EDITOR

HOLLY M. HOLMES, MD
Assistant Professor, Department of General Internal Medicine, The University of Texas
MD Anderson Cancer Center, Houston, Texas

AUTHORS

CHRISTINA L. BELL, MD, MS
Assistant Professor in Geriatric Medicine, The John A. Hartford Center of Excellence in
Geriatrics, Department of Geriatric Medicine, John A. Burns School of Medicine,
University of Hawaii, Honolulu, Hawaii

MARIE C. BRADLEY, PhD, MPharm, MPSI, MPSNI
HRB Centre for Primary Care Research, Royal College of Surgeons in Ireland (RCSI),
Division of Population Health Science, Dublin, Ireland; School of Pharmacy, Queen's
University Belfast, Belfast, Northern Ireland, United Kingdom

BARBARA CLYNE, BSocSC, MSocSC
HRB Centre for Primary Care Research, Royal College of Surgeons in Ireland (RCSI),
Division of Population Health Science, Dublin, Ireland

DAVID G. LE COUTEUR, MBBS, PhD
Sydney Medical School, University of Sydney; Centre for Education and Research on
Ageing, Concord Hospital; and ANZAC Medical Research Institute, Concord Hospital
and University of Sydney, Concord NSW, Australia

TOM FAHEY, MSc, MD, DCH, Dobs, MEdCert, MFPH, FRCGP
HRB Centre for Primary Care Research, Royal College of Surgeons in Ireland (RCSI),
Division of Population Health Science, Dublin, Ireland

STEPHEN P. FITZGERALD, MB, BS, FRACP
Consultant Physician, Department of Internal Medicine, Royal Adelaide Hospital,
Adelaide, South Australia, Australia

WALID F. GELLAD, MD, MPH
Center for Health Equity Research and Promotion, Veterans Affairs Pittsburgh
Healthcare System; Assistant Professor, Department of Medicine (General Medicine),
School of Medicine, University of Pittsburgh and RAND Health, Pittsburgh, Pennsylvania

JANE GIVENS, MD, MSCE
Assistant Professor of Medicine, Division of Gerontology, Beth Israel Deaconess
Medical Center; Hebrew SeniorLife Institute for Aging Research, Boston, Massachusetts

DANIJELA GNJIDIC, PhD, MPH
Departments of Clinical Pharmacology and Aged Care, Royal North Shore Hospital, St
Leonards NSW; Sydney Medical School, University of Sydney; and Centre for Education
and Research on Ageing, Concord Hospital, Concord NSW, Australia

MURTHY GOKULA, MD
Assistant Professor/Program Director, Geriatric Medicine Fellowship Program,
St. Luke's Hospital/University of Toledo, Maumee, Ohio

EMILY R. HAJJAR, PharmD, BCPS, BCACP, CGP
Associate Professor, Jefferson School of Pharmacy, Thomas Jefferson University,
Philadelphia, Pennsylvania

SARAH N. HILMER, MBBS, PhD
Departments of Clinical Pharmacology and Aged Care, Royal North Shore Hospital, St
Leonards NSW; and Sydney Medical School, University of Sydney, NWS, Australia

HOLLY M. HOLMES, MD
Assistant Professor, Department of General Internal Medicine, University of Texas MD
Anderson Cancer Center, Houston, Texas

BO HOVSTADIUS, PhD
eHealth Institute; School of Natural Sciences, Linnaeus University, Kalmar, Sweden

CARMEL HUGHES, PhD, MRPharmS, MPSNI
School of Pharmacy, Queen's University Belfast, Belfast, Northern Ireland, United
Kingdom

MICHIKO INABA, MD, PhD
Assistant Professor in Geriatric Medicine, The John A. Hartford Center of Excellence in
Geriatrics, Department of Geriatric Medicine, John A. Burns School of Medicine,
University of Hawaii, Honolulu, Hawaii

LISA KOULADJIAN, BMedSc (Hons), MPharm
Departments of Clinical Pharmacology and Aged Care, Royal North Shore Hospital, St
Leonards NSW, Australia

KATE L. LAPANE, PhD
Virginia Commonwealth University, Richmond, Virginia

ZACHARY A. MARCUM, PharmD, MS
Assistant Professor, Department of Medicine (Geriatrics), School of Medicine, University
of Pittsburgh, Pittsburgh, Pennsylvania

KAMAL H. MASAKI, MD
Professor in Geriatric Medicine, The John A. Hartford Center of Excellence in Geriatrics,
Department of Geriatric Medicine, John A. Burns School of Medicine, University of
Hawaii, Honolulu, Hawaii

MARY LYNN MCPHERSON, PharmD, BPCS, CPE
Professor and Vice Chair, Department of Pharmacy Practice and Science, University of
Maryland School of Pharmacy, Baltimore, Maryland

GÖRAN PETERSSON, MD, PhD
Professor, eHealth Institute; School of Health and Caring Sciences, Linnaeus University,
Kalmar, Sweden

RAVI P. RUBERU, MB, BS, PhD
Clinical Lecturer, Faculty of Medicine; Senior Registrar in Geriatric and Rehabilitation
Medicine, Royal Adelaide Hospital, Adelaide, South Australia, Australia

LEAH CHURCH SERA, PharmD
Pain and Palliative Care Resident, Department of Pharmacy Practice and Science,
University of Maryland School of Pharmacy, Baltimore, Maryland

BHAVIK M. SHAH, PharmD, BCPS
Assistant Professor, Jefferson School of Pharmacy, Thomas Jefferson University, Philadelphia, Pennsylvania

BRUCE K. TAMURA, MD
Assistant Professor in Geriatric Medicine, The John A. Hartford Center of Excellence in Geriatrics, Department of Geriatric Medicine, John A. Burns School of Medicine, University of Hawaii, Honolulu, Hawaii

JENNIFER TJIA, MD, MSCE
Assistant Professor of Medicine, Division of Geriatric Medicine, University of Massachusetts Medical School, Worcester, Massachusetts

Contents

of great importance in reducing unnecessary or burdensome medications. This article reviews the ethical principles for medication discontinuation, discusses in a case-based format on how to apply an ethical framework to prescribing challenges, and offers practical considerations for medication discontinuation.

Knowledge of the physiologic changes associated with aging is vital to providing optimal pharmaceutical care to geriatric patients. The absorption, distribution, metabolism, and excretion of medications are affected to varying extents by the normal aging process and by disease states commonly associated with increasing age. Additionally, altered pharmacodynamics in the elderly—the magnitude of a drug's pharmacologic effect—may increase the risk for adverse drug effects in this population. The altered action and disposition of drugs in the elderly patient should be taken into account by health care professionals to improve adherence, provide appropriate counseling, minimize side effects, and reduce medication errors.

Polypharmacy and medication adherence present a unique challenge for the older adult, their caregiver(s), and the health care team. There appears to be an association in the literature between polypharmacy and poorer medication adherence in older adults. However, the heterogeneity of how adherence is defined in the literature limits the certainty of this conclusion. Nonetheless, improving medication adherence to maximize the therapeutic benefit of pharmacotherapy remains a cornerstone of geriatric care. We discuss strategies for limiting polypharmacy and improving adherence and suggest ideas for future research focused on identifying and translating safe and effective interventions to improve adherence into routine clinical practice.

Prescribing appropriate medications for older people is challenging. Older people tend to have multiple conditions, require multiple drug treatments, experience increased sensitivity to medications due to physiological age related changes, and consequently, are vulnerable to inappropriate prescribing, polypharmacy and adverse drug events. This review provides an overview of current evidence in relation to electronic prescribing and other technologies, particularly computerized decision support systems, in reducing inappropriate medication use in the prescribing stage. We discuss the concepts of inappropriate prescribing, polypharmacy, and health information technology and summarize the evidence in light of the challenges of implementing technology into practice.

Murthy Gokula and Holly M. Holmes

Polypharmacy and inappropriate medication use are prevalent problems in older persons. Although multidimensional interventions may help to improve prescribing, such models of care may not routinely be available to the busy clinician. We briefly present a number of commonly used tools for medication review that are designed to identify and reduce inappropriate medication use and polypharmacy.

THE CLINICS ARE NOW AVAILABLE ONLINE!

Access your subscription at:
www.theclinics.com

Preface

Polypharmacy

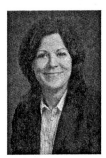

Holly M. Holmes, MD
Guest Editor

Polypharmacy has been a persistent issue in caring for older persons. The use of excess numbers of medications is burdensome in many ways to older patients, increasing the risk for adverse drug reactions, inappropriate medication use, and health care costs. Defining polypharmacy, developing ways to identify it in clinical and research settings, intervening to reduce it, and understanding the consequences of polypharmacy all continue to be controversial areas for discussion among health care providers who are focused on improving the quality of care for older persons.

In this special issue of *Clinics in Geriatric Medicine* devoted to polypharmacy, multiple authors have covered the breadth of the diverse issues related to polypharmacy. We have attempted to provide meaningful, evidence-based definitions of what constitutes polypharmacy. We have focused on specific situations and populations in which polypharmacy is especially problematic, namely, persons with multiple comorbid conditions and patients in long-term care. We have also devoted a number of articles to methods, tools, and outcomes related to medication discontinuation, including a case-based discussion of ethical issues. Finally, specific articles review topics integrally related to polypharmacy, including age-related changes in pharmacokinetics and medication adherence.

As the older population continues to grow, managing a complex profile of comorbid conditions and multiple medications will become an increasing challenge for medical providers engaged in the care of older persons. The contributions of the authors to this special issue provide an excellent framework for clinical challenges and research

Clin Geriatr Med 28 (2012) xiii–xiv
doi:10.1016/j.cger.2012.01.012
geriatric.theclinics.com

initiatives, and we hope this issue will stimulate critical further dialogue about the growing problem of polypharmacy.

Holly M. Holmes, MD
Department of General Internal Medicine
The University of Texas MD Anderson Cancer Center
1400 Pressler, Unit 1465, FCT 13.5028
Houston, TX 77030, USA

E-mail address:
hholmes@mdanderson.org

Factors Leading to Excessive Polypharmacy

Bo Hovstadius, PhD[a,b,]*, Göran Petersson, MD, PhD[a,c]

KEYWORDS

- Polypharmacy • Risk factors • Elderly • Morbidity

Polypharmacy can be defined as the concurrent use of many different drugs. Polypharmacy can also be defined as the excessive use of drugs, for example the use of a number of drugs in excess of that which is clinically indicated, or the use of an excessive number of inappropriate drugs.[1]

Polypharmacy is intended to comprise all of the individual's concomitantly consumed drugs, regardless if they are described as chronic medication, required medication, or short-term drugs. Polypharmacy should be seen to include all types of medications, in other words prescription drugs, over-the-counter (OTC) drugs, complementary and alternative medicine (CAM), and dietary supplements.

Prescription drugs are seen to compose the basis of studies concerning drug utilization. Physicians, researchers, and patients often consider prescription drugs as being more potent and important than other types of drugs; for example, 40% of the population believe that OTC drugs are too weak to cause any real harm.[2] Furthermore, in studies of drug utilization, the focus is often on chronically applied drugs.

OTC drugs are not always included in studies of patients' drug use. Normally, sales data for OTC drugs refer only to the total population. Consequently, our knowledge of the use of OTC drugs in different gender, age, or health strata is often based on interview studies, the results of which are extrapolated to general assumptions of the use of OTC drugs in entire populations. In spite of the fact that the use of dietary supplements and CAM is extensive,[3] and in spite of the fact that these substances may interact with the individual's prescribed drugs, they are usually excluded in studies of drug use.

NUMBER OF MEDICATIONS

As a threshold for polypharmacy, two or more,[4,5] three or more,[6] four or more,[7] five or more,[8–13] six or more,[4,14] seven or more,[15] nine or more,[16,17] and 10 or

[a] eHealth Institute, Linnaeus University, Bredbandet 1, PO SE-391 82 Kalmar, Sweden
[b] School of Natural Sciences, Linnaeus University, Barlastgatan 11, PO SE-391 82 Kalmar, Sweden
[c] School of Health and Caring Sciences, Linnaeus University, Stagneliusgatan 14, PO SE-391 82 Kalmar, Sweden
* Corresponding author. PwC, PO Box 179, SE-751 04 Uppsala, Sweden.
E-mail address: bo.hovstadius@pwc.se

Clin Geriatr Med 28 (2012) 159–172
doi:10.1016/j.cger.2012.01.001
0749-0690/12/$ – see front matter © 2012 Published by Elsevier Inc.

geriatric.theclinics.com

more[9,15,18,19] drugs has been used. The majority of studies have applied five or more (prescribed) drugs as the threshold for polypharmacy.[9,11,20] Over time, as the number of concomitantly used drugs has consistently increased, the focus on the number of drugs has changed. Early studies of polypharmacy focused on the concurrent use of two, three, or four drugs. In 1997, Bjerrum and colleagues[8] defined the concomitant use of two to four drugs as "minor" polypharmacy and the use of five or more drugs as "major" polypharmacy. In 2000, Veehof and colleagues[4] classified two to three drugs as "minor," four to five drugs as "moderate," and six or more as "major" polypharmacy. In 2011, Jyrkkä and colleagues[21] categorized zero to five drugs as "no polypharmacy," six to nine drugs as "polypharmacy," and 10 or more drugs as "excessive polypharmacy."[21,22] In current studies, the use of five or more drugs has become a form of standard cutoff for clinically relevant polypharmacy, but the scale has also been extended and "excessive polypharmacy," defined as the concurrent use of 10 or more drugs, is also studied.[18,19,23]

Whether any given number of drugs is relevant as a measure of polypharmacy from a clinical perspective is under debate,[11,24] and researchers have argued that selecting appropriate limits for the number of medications may be counterproductive in populations with multiple comorbidities.[23] Even if today there is a consensus that 10 or more drugs is considered to be the standard definition of excessive polypharmacy, in the following discussion the authors refer to excessive polypharmacy as implying the use of more drugs than are clinically indicated and not to a specific number of drugs. Consequently, the authors review factors that in studies have been presented as resulting in the excessive use of medications, and not only if they result in the use of 10 or more drugs.

OCCURRENCE OF POLYPHARMACY

The observed occurrence of polypharmacy in a given population is dependent on the true occurrence and on the measurement that has been applied in the estimates. Some studies apply a point prevalence approach and specify the number of individuals of different ages and gender having used a drug during a certain day or week. Other studies focus on the use of different types of drugs during longer study periods, for example 2 to 12 months. In addition to the large variations in the time periods, studies of polypharmacy have been conducted on the basis of different definitions, for example more than two, three, four, five, six seven, nine or 10 drugs. Furthermore, studies have included patients from different settings, for example outpatients, patients admitted to hospitals or nursing homes, patients with different ages, or patients with different medical conditions, for example, psychiatric diseases. The majority of the studies have been conducted in small samples of elderly individuals, but some have been population-based. Because of the large variation in study settings, there is also a large variation in results regarding the prevalence of polypharmacy. Furthermore, there are also large differences in the types of drugs included in the different studies. As mentioned earlier, CAM and dietary supplements are seldom included. Many studies also focus on drugs for chronic therapy and therefore exclude as-needed drugs, topical drugs, and drugs for short time use, such as antibacterials.[7,25,26] Other studies include only governmental subsidized medication.[8,9] Consequently, the prevalence of polypharmacy varies according to the definition of polypharmacy. In 1998 and 1999, a total of 25% of the US population aged 18 and above had taken five or more drugs a week (prescription drugs, OTC drugs, CAM, and dietary supplements) and 5% had taken 10 or more. Of women aged 65 and over, 57% had taken five or more, and 12% had taken 10 or more drugs.[27] In 2005 and 2006, a total of 29% of all individuals in the US aged 57 through 85

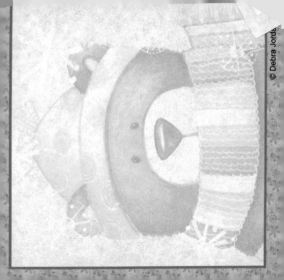

regularly used at least five prescription drugs. Among prescription drug users, the concurrent use of OTC drugs was 46%, and there was 52% concurrent use of dietary supplements.[28] To conclude, the knowledge regarding individual use of prescription drugs seems to be fairly good, but there is little knowledge as regards the individual use of OTC drugs, CAM, and dietary supplements. Consequently, there is also a lack of knowledge as regards patients' combinations of the different types of medications, for example how many individuals of different ages and gender combine prescription drugs, OTC drugs, and CAM in conjunction with, or without, dietary supplements.

If this pattern expands to various groups of individuals with polypharmacy, the uncertainty as regards the prevalence of different drug combinations becomes even more notable. The large variations between studies regarding age groups, cutoffs, study periods, and types of medications make it difficult to compare the results.

CONSEQUENCES OF POLYPHARMACY

The use of medication is intended to have a beneficial effect on patient health and the quality of life. However, the use of medications might be counterproductive, in other words, they do not have only beneficial effects on humans. The use of medications, and especially the use of multiple medications, polypharmacy, is also associated with the risk of negative consequences.

Adverse Drug Reaction

Many medications may result in an adverse drug reaction (ADR).[29] Whether an ADR will occur and how severe it will be varies with regard to the drug in question and the individual's specific circumstances. ADR represents a substantial proportion of all admissions to hospitals and a substantial proportion of the health care costs. Approximately 5% to 6% of hospital admissions are associated with ADRs,[30] and as much as 12% in older patients.[5] Deaths caused by ADRs are estimated to be the fourth most common death cause in US hospitals.[31] In Norway, 18% of deaths in departments of internal medicine are reported to be caused by ADRs.[32] In Sweden, approximately 3.3% of all deaths are caused by ADRs.[33]

Interactions

The effect of a medication can be influenced by other medications that the individual may be taking (drug-drug interaction), food, beverages, or supplements that the individual is consuming (nutrient-drug interactions), and another disease (disease-drug interactions).

Drug-drug interactions include all types of drugs, prescription drugs, OTC drugs, and CAM. Theoretically, the risk for drug-drug interactions increases exponentially with the number of ingested drugs[34,35]; for example, for five drugs there are 10 possible one-to-one interactions, for 10 drugs there are 45, and for 15 drugs there are 105 possible interactions. Also, a strong association between the number of dispensed drugs and the probability of potential interactions has been demonstrated.[36]

Nutrient-drug interactions include herbs and vitamins, which can interact with drug-metabolizing enzymes. One well-known example is St John's wort, which can interact with several important medications.[37] Colas, coffee, and chocolate containing caffeine are known to possibly interact with certain antibiotics, and grapefruit juice and alcohol are also known to interact with certain drugs.[37]

Disease-drug interactions occur when a disease worsens because of a drug pre-scribed for a reason other than to treat that disease. Potential disease-drug interactions are common in hospitalized elderly patients.[38] To prevent disease-drug interactions, there are clinical guidelines regarding drugs and drug classes that the physician should not prescribe to patients with certain diseases.[39]

Nonadherence to Drug Therapy

Patients' adherence to drug therapy is essential in optimizing the disease treatment, and nonadherence is associated with poor health outcomes.[40–42] Polypharmacy is commonly associated with nonadherence, and it is assumed that the prevalence of nonadherence increases with an increasing number of prescribed drugs.[8,35,43–45]

Inappropriate Prescribing

There are several criteria for classifying inappropriate prescriptions, almost all with the focus on elderly individuals' drug use; for example, Beers criteria,[46] Improving Prescribing in the Elderly Tool (IPET),[47] Screening Tool to Alert doctors to Right Treatment (START),[48] Screening Tool of Older persons' Potentially inappropriate Prescriptions (STOPP),[49] McLeod criteria,[50] and the Medication Appropriateness Index (MAI).[51] Furthermore, some studies apply a combination of several of the more well-known criteria.[52]

According to Beers' criteria, the prescription of potentially inappropriate medica-tions to older people is highly prevalent in the United States and Europe, ranging from 12% in community-dwelling elderly to 40% in nursing home residents.[53] Moreover, the proportion of inappropriate medications has been shown to increase with the number of drugs prescribed.[35,54]

Underuse of Medication

The use of many different drugs is often associated with inappropriate medication use and underuse. In the United States, a total of 64% of outpatients aged 65 and older with five or more medications did not use one or more indicated medications.[54]

In the Netherlands, a relationship between polypharmacy (patients with five or more drugs) and underprescribing is also noted. Of patients with polypharmacy, 43% were undertreated in comparison with 14% of patients using four medicines or less, and the probability of underprescribing increased with the number of drugs.[13] It seems to be a paradox, that the risk of underprescribing increases with the use of an increasing number of drugs.[55]

FACTORS ASSOCIATED WITH POLYPHARMACY

The large majority of studies concerning polypharmacy deal with its potential negative effects, for example ADR, interactions, and increasing nonadherence to drug therapy. Some studies focus on testing the effect of interventions and are aimed at reducing the number of drugs taken by patients or at adjusting inappropriate multiple medication therapy. The many and various factors possibly causing polypharmacy have not been studied to the same extent as the consequences of polypharmacy. A large number of varying conditions and factors have been demonstrated to be associated with polypharmacy, but causality has not always been explicitly deter-mined (**Box 1**).

Factors Related to the Health Care System

Certain factors leading to excessive polypharmacy are associated with the develop-ment of society and health care services. Ongoing medical developments have

---

Box 1
Factors associated with polypharmacy

Factors related to the health care system

  Increased life expectancy

  Development of new therapies and technologies

  Increased use of preventive strategies

Factors related to patients

  Age

  Gender

  Race/ethnicity

  Socioeconomic status

  Clinical conditions

  Medical therapy

  Behavior

Factors related to physicians

  Premises

  Medical guidelines

  Prescribing habits

  Behavior

The interaction between patient and physician

---

contributed to increasing the overall length of life. The number of elderly individuals with chronic diseases has increased because of this increase.[14,56] Medical developments have successively increased the number of conditions that can be treated[11,19] and have also further developed existing therapies.[14,19,43,57–60] In addition, the increased use of primary and secondary preventive prescribing strategies has contributed to increasing drug use and can, therefore, be seen as a risk factor in terms of excessive polypharmacy.[43]

The ongoing development of new medications and the general development of society have also resulted in an increasing use of health care services.[14] A negative consequence of this development is hospitalization, which is a known risk factor for excessive polypharmacy.[4,15]

PATIENT-RELATED FACTORS
Age

Even if the majority of individuals with polypharmacy are less than 70 years of age,[61] a number of studies show that the average number of drugs increases with increasing age, because age is one of the most common risk factors for excessive polypharmacy.[4,5,19,35,55,61–64] With increasing age the prevalence of diseases increases, resulting in a greater proportion of prescribed drugs.[35] In an entire national population, the prevalence of polypharmacy increased from 18.4% in the age group 40 to 49 years to 30.2% in 50 to 59 years, to 42.3% in 60 to 69 years, to 62.4% in 70 to 79 years, to 75.1% in 80 to 89 years, and to 77.7% in the age group 90 years and above.[61] The average number of dispensed prescription drugs per individual during a 12-month study period was 7.9 (median 7, quartile [Q] 1–Q3 4–11) for patients 70 to 79 years, 9.3 (median 8, Q1–Q3 5–13) for 80 to 89 years, and 9.7 (median 9, Q1–Q3 6–13) for 90 years and above.[61]

Gender

Generally, women take more medications than men, with a higher prevalence of polypharmacy than for men. Therefore, several studies have defined gender as a risk factor for excessive polypharmacy.[5,9,14,62,63,65] In higher age categories, the relative risk for polypharmacy for women versus men levels out, and no general gender factor for elderly individuals can be identified.[9,66,67] When studied in an entire national population, the relative risk for women versus men to receive five or more drugs is found to be 3.1 in the age group 20 to 29, followed by a successive decrease to 1.1 in the age group 70 years and above.[61]

Race/Ethnicity

The overall prevalence of drug use varies somewhat according to race/ethnicity, for example in the United States, from 84% for white Americans to 57% among Asian/Pacific Islanders.[27] Therefore, it can be assumed that race/ethnicity also might represent a general risk factor for excessive polypharmacy.

Socioeconomic Factors

Individuals' use of drugs and the risk of excessive polypharmacy is also associated with patients' socioeconomic status. However, some conflicting results have been presented. Less wealthy individuals have a greater risk of experiencing polypharmacy.[68] Still, good insurance coverage has been shown to be associated with excessive polypharmacy.[5,65] The patient's education level might also represent a risk factor for excessive polypharmacy. Again, there are some conflicting results. Certain studies claim that less educated individuals have an increasing risk of excessive polypharmacy,[5,10,18] whereas other studies have found no association between excessive polypharmacy and educational level.[14,20,69]

CLINICAL CONDITIONS

Factors associated with patients' clinical conditions are common among studies of polypharmacy. Poor health,[5,65] chronic conditions,[60,65,67] and varying specific diseases are demonstrated to be linked with polypharmacy[5,25]; for example, cardiovascular diseases (odds ratio [OR] 4.5), anemia (OR 4.1) and respiratory diseases (OR 3.6).[9] Factors that are associated with both polypharmacy (PP) and excessive polypharmacy (EPP) include poor self-reported health (PP: OR 2.15 and EPP: OR 6.02), diabetes mellitus (PP: OR 2.28 and EPP: OR 2.07), depression (PP: OR 2.13 and EPP: OR 2.93), pain (PP: OR 2.69 and EPP: OR 2.74), heart disease (PP: OR 2.51 and EPP: OR 4.63), and obstructive pulmonary disease (PP: OR 2.79 and EPP: OR 6.82).[63] In a review of nine studies, depression, hypertension, anemia, asthma, angina, diverticulosis, osteoarthritis, gout, and diabetes mellitus are associated with polypharmacy.[5]

Also, poor self-perceived health and poor life satisfaction are believed to represent risk factors for excessive polypharmacy.[14,25,63,67] Other patient conditions associated with excessive polypharmacy include declining nutrition, ability to function, and cognitive capacity.[21] Multiple diseases or multiple symptoms are common risk factors, with a strong correlation demonstrated between the number of diseases and the number of drugs used.[5,19,35,62,67,70–74]

Medical Therapy

Studies concerning the type of drugs associated with excessive polypharmacy show a large variation, and the results are often difficult to compare because of different study settings. Cardiovascular medication is often on the top of the list.[9] In a study of an entire national population, the prevalence of the five most frequently dispensed drug groups, for the 2.2 million individuals with five or more dispensed prescription drugs, were antibacterials (48.2%), analgesics (40.3%), psycholeptics (35.9%), antithrombotic agents (33.4%), and beta blocking agents (31.7%).[75]

Patient Behavior

Another perspective as regards the risk of excessive polypharmacy is focused on patient behavior. Regardless of premises and conditions, patient self-medication is shown to represent an independent risk factor for excessive polypharmacy.[6,27,28,35,71,76–79] Many patients ingest large amounts of different types of medication: prescribed, OTC, CAM, and so forth. One-third of 75-year olds living in their own home used three or more OTC drugs each day.[6] General practitioners' (GPs') knowledge concerning their patient total drug use has been shown to be limited. In one study, a total of 37% of the patients took prescription drugs without their GP's knowledge.[77] Another study reported a situation in which 24% of all the prescribed drugs were used without the GPs' knowledge.[6] This situation is problematic and is not improved by the fact that GPs often exclude all but chronic medications in their review of the patient's medication list.[80]

Another complicating factor concerning patients' behavior is the borrowing and sharing of prescribed drugs by patients.[35,76,81,82] Older people often receive medication from relatives or friends but they do not perceive this medication as their own, and therefore they seldom mention these drugs in any medical examination.[79]

PHYSICIAN-RELATED FACTORS

The second most important group of risk factors for patients to be exposed to excessive polypharmacy is related to the physician, because prescribed drugs account for the majority of all medication used by the patients, excluding the patients' self-medication of OTC, CAM, and dietary supplements.

Physician Practice Environment

The prevalence of polypharmacy between comparable practices varies from a fourfold variation in one study including 730 GPs[83] and a sixfold variation in another study including 173 GPs.[84] In the latter study, six predictors related to the physicians explained 56% of the variations. According to Bjerrum and colleagues,[84] polypharmacy was related a low number of listed patients, a high workload, a low rate of admission to hospital, a high practice prescribing rate, and a high average number of different prescribed medications. Lack of time and high workload are also seen as reasons for medications remaining in the patients' records longer than necessary.[80] Physicians' education and competence are of vital importance to the patients' drug therapy. Lack of accurate education and competence is an obvious risk factor for excessive polypharmacy.[58,74,85,86] The prevalence of polypharmacy is lower for female than for male GPs (36 per 1000 listed versus 46 per 1000 listed) but is not associated with the age of the physician or the number of years in general practice.[84]

Medical Guidelines

Medical guidelines are intended to support physicians in their choice of drug therapy. However, guidelines can be an important risk factor for excessive polypharmacy, especially for patients with multiple diseases.[19,55,58,80,87–89] Guidelines normally focus on one particular disease and can, therefore, serve as "medical generators" for patients with multiple diseases. GPs trust them but find them difficult to apply to patients with multiple diseases.[80] Guidelines might contribute to explaining the age trend in development of excessive polypharmacy, because older patients are exposed more often to several diseases, and therefore more frequently receive several additional drugs. Physicians perceive other demands that are associated with excessive polypharmacy, for example employer pressure or pressure from colleagues to provide multiple medications and to shorten hospital days.[60]

Prescribing Habits

The active process conducted by a physician leading to excessive polypharmacy is the prescribing of a given drug to the patient. The belief and dominant perception that diseases should be treated with drugs, and that a visit to the physician should end with a prescription, contribute to excessive polypharmacy.[35,60,70]

When reviewing patients' medication lists, many patients are found to be prescribed unnecessary drugs,[5,58,76,90] and some of these drugs are therapeutic duplicates.[5,76] Furthermore, the proportion of inappropriate medications has been shown to increase with the number of drugs.[17,35,54]

Excessive polypharmacy is also associated with the risk of "medical cascade" effects or "prescribing cascades." The prescribing cascades are initiated when an ADR is misinterpreted as a new medical condition, with the subsequent new prescription of additional drugs. Thereafter, a new adverse reaction may occur that can be mistakenly diagnosed as a new medical problem, which can lead to an additional number of prescriptions of medications.[35,73,76,87,91]

Physician Behavior

Risk factors for patients experiencing excessive polypharmacy include what the physician fails to do; in other words, if the physician does not take a proper medical review.[19,70,92] It is of vital importance that the communication and coordination between GPs and hospital doctors is accurate, because such a lack of communication is a risk factor of excessive polypharmacy.[6,55,71,80] Problems occur when physicians provide unclear instructions in trying to stop the use of a certain medication[35,80] or when imprecise diagnoses are provided.[58] As mentioned earlier, medical guidelines can be perceived as medical generators, but the physician's skepticism as regards following guidelines can also be regarded to represent a risk factor for excessive polypharmacy; for example, when psychiatrists mistrust research and new recommendations of optimal antipsychotic treatment and stick to old prescribing traditions with polypharmacy and excessive dosing.[93]

FACTORS RELATED TO THE INTERACTION BETWEEN PATIENT AND PHYSICIAN

A good interaction between the patient and the physician is essential to good medical treatment. Patients' adherence to drug therapy depends, among many other things, on the confidence between patient and physician. The interaction between patient and physician has been a subject identified as a possible factor leading to excessive polypharmacy. Patients who fail to review their entire medication list for their physician are at a greater risk of excessive polypharmacy.[70,77] The lack of personnel continuity among different health services providers seems to be a risk factor for excessive polypharmacy, because a patient with multiple health providers, multiple prescribers, or multiple pharmacies is also at greater risk of experiencing excessive polypharmacy.[4,5,35,55,70,72,80,94]

Patients' expectations of receiving prescriptions for multiple medications at a visit to the doctor are associated with increasing multiple drug use.[4] The patients' demands or requests on doctors for multiple medications are also recognized as a factor that can lead to excessive drug use and the development of excessive polypharmacy.[4,35,60,74,80,95] In addition, disagreements between patients and physicians about treatment are seen as a factor that can lead to excessive polypharmacy.[25]

SUMMARY

There are numerous risk factors for patients to develop excessive polypharmacy. The most prominent risk factors are associated with sociodemographics and the patients' conditions. Risk factors associated with patient behavior, such as patient's self-medication with all types of medications, have not been observed to the same extent but might be at the same level of importance for patients developing excessive polypharmacy.

Risk factors related to physicians, and the interaction between patient and physician, are studied to a much lesser extent. The few studies conducted regarding the large variation in physicians' individual prescribing practices, in terms of polypharmacy, add another perspective to the complexity of the area. Interventions aiming to improve communication between GP and hospital specialist, to create support systems for medical reviews that include all patients' medications, and to improve the knowledge of multiple prescribing might have the largest potential to better manage excessive polypharmacy.

REFERENCES

1. WHO Centre for Health Development. A glossary of terms for community health care and services for older persons. Ageing and health technical report, vol 5. Geneva (Switzerland): World Health Organization; 2004.
2. Roumie CL, Griffin MR. Over-the-counter analgesics in older adults: a call for improved labelling and consumer education. Drugs Aging 2004;21(8):485–98.
3. Barnes PM, Bloom B, Nahin RL. Complementary and alternative medicine use among adults and children: United States, 2007. Natl Health Stat Report 2008;(12):1–23.
4. Veehof L, Stewart R, Haaijer-Ruskamp F, et al. The development of polypharmacy. A longitudinal study. Fam Pract 2000;17(3):261–7.
5. Hajjar ER, Cafiero AC, Hanlon JT. Polypharmacy in elderly patients. Am J Geriatr Pharmacother 2007;5(4):345–51.
6. Barat I, Andreasen F, Damsgaard EM. The consumption of drugs by 75-year-old individuals living in their own homes. Eur J Clin Pharmacol 2000;56(6-7):501–9.
7. Denneboom W, Dautzenberg MG, Grol R, et al. Analysis of polypharmacy in older patients in primary care using a multidisciplinary expert panel. Br J Gen Pract 2006;56(528):504–10.
8. Bjerrum L, Rosholm JU, Hallas J, et al. Methods for estimating the occurrence of polypharmacy by means of a prescription database. Eur J Clin Pharmacol 1997;53(1): 7–11.
9. Bjerrum L, Sogaard J, Hallas J, et al. Polypharmacy: correlations with sex, age and drug regimen. A prescription database study. Eur J Clin Pharmacol 1998;54(3):197–202.
10. Haider SI, Johnell K, Thorslund M, et al. Trends in polypharmacy and potential drug-drug interactions across educational groups in elderly patients in Sweden for the period 1992 - 2002. Int J Clin Pharmacol Ther 2007;45(12):643–53.

11. Viktil KK, Blix HS, Moger TA, Reikvam A. Polypharmacy as commonly defined is an indicator of limited value in the assessment of drug-related problems. Br J Clin Pharmacol 2007;63(2):187–95.

12. Linton A, Garber M, Fagan NK, et al. Examination of multiple medication use among TRICARE beneficiaries aged 65 years and older. J Manag Care Pharm 2007;13(2): 155–62.

13. Kuijpers MA, van Marum RJ, Egberts AC, et al. Relationship between polypharmacy and underprescribing. Br J Clin Pharmacol 2008;65(1):130–3.

14. Linjakumpu T, Hartikainen S, Klaukka T, et al. Use of medications and polypharmacy are increasing among the elderly. J Clin Epidemiol 2002;55(8):809–17.

15. Flaherty JH, Perry HM 3rd, Lynchard GS, et al. Polypharmacy and hospitalization among older home care patients. J Gerontol A Biol Sci Med Sci 2000;55(10):M554–9.

16. Nguyen JK, Fouts MM, Kotabe SE, et al. Polypharmacy as a risk factor for adverse drug reactions in geriatric nursing home residents. Am J Geriatr Pharmacother 2006;4(1):36–41.

17. Fialova D, Topinkova E, Gambassi G, et al. Potentially inappropriate medication use among elderly home care patients in Europe. JAMA 2005;293(11):1348–58.

18. Haider SI, Johnell K, Weitoft GR, et al. The influence of educational level on polypharmacy and inappropriate drug use: a register-based study of more than 600,000 older people. J Am Geriatr Soc 2009;57(1):62–9.

19. Jyrkka J, Vartiainen L, Hartikainen S, et al. Increasing use of medicines in elderly persons: a five-year follow-up of the Kuopio 75+Study. Eur J Clin Pharmacol 2006;62(2):151–8.

20. Haider SI, Johnell K, Thorslund M, et al. Analysis of the association between polypharmacy and socioeconomic position among elderly aged >/=77 years in Sweden. Clin Ther 2008;30(2):419–27.

21. Jyrkka J, Enlund H, Lavikainen P, et al. Association of polypharmacy with nutritional status, functional ability and cognitive capacity over a three-year period in an elderly population. Pharmacoepidemiol Drug Saf 2011;20(5):514–22.

22. Jyrkkä J, Enlund H, Korhonen MJ, et al. Polypharmacy status as an indicator of mortality in an elderly population. Drugs Aging 2009;26(12):1039–48.

23. Fulton MM, Allen ER. Polypharmacy in the elderly: a literature review. J Am Acad Nurse Pract 2005;17(4):123–32.

24. Aronson JK. Polypharmacy, appropriate and inappropriate. Br J Gen Pract 2006; 56(528):484–5.

25. Junius-Walker U, Theile G, Hummers-Pradier E. Prevalence and predictors of polypharmacy among older primary care patients in Germany. Fam Pract 2007;24(1):14–9.

26. Johnell K, Fastbom J, Rosen M, et al. Inappropriate drug use in the elderly: a nationwide register-based study. Ann Pharmacother 2007;41(7):1243–8.

27. Kaufman DW, Kelly JP, Rosenberg L, et al. Recent patterns of medication use in the ambulatory adult population of the United States: the Slone survey. JAMA 2002; 287(3):337–44.

28. Qato DM, Alexander GC, Conti RM, et al. Use of prescription and over-the-counter medications and dietary supplements among older adults in the United States. JAMA 2008;300(24):2867–78.

29. International drug monitoring. The role of national centres. WHO technical report No 498. Geneva (Switzerland): World Health Organization; 1972.

30. Kongkaew C, Noyce PR, Ashcroft DM. Hospital admissions associated with adverse drug reactions: a systematic review of prospective observational studies. Ann Pharmacother 2008;42(7):1017–25.

31. Lazarou J, Pomeranz BH, Corey PN. Incidence of adverse drug reactions in hospitalized patients: a meta-analysis of prospective studies. JAMA 1998;279(15):1200–5.
32. Ebbesen J, Buajordet I, Erikssen J, et al. Drug-related deaths in a department of internal medicine. Arch Intern Med 2001;161(19):2317–23.
33. Jonsson AK, Hakkarainen KM, Spigset O, et al. Preventable drug related mortality in a Swedish population. Pharmacoepidemiol Drug Saf 2010;19(2):211–5.
34. Cadieux RJ. Drug interactions in the elderly. How multiple drug use increases risk exponentially. Postgrad Med 1989;86(8):179–86.
35. Colley CA, Lucas LM. Polypharmacy: the cure becomes the disease. J Gen Intern Med 1993;8(5):278–83.
36. Johnell K, Klarin I. The relationship between number of drugs and potential drug-drug interactions in the elderly: a study of over 600,000 elderly patients from the Swedish Prescribed Drug Register. Drug Saf 2007;30(10):911–8.
37. Sjöqvist, F. Interaktion mellan läkemedel [Drug-drug interactions]. FASS 2012:11–8. The Swedish Association of the Pharmaceutical Industry [in Swedish].
38. Lindblad CI, Artz MB, Pieper CF, et al. Potential drug-disease interactions in frail, hospitalized elderly veterans. Ann Pharmacother 2005;39(3):412–7.
39. Hanlon JT, Schmader KE, Ruby CM, et al. Suboptimal prescribing in older inpatients and outpatients. J Am Geriatr Soc 2001;49(2):200–9.
40. Simpson SH, Eurich DT, Majumdar SR, et al. A meta-analysis of the association between adherence to drug therapy and mortality. BMJ 2006;333(7557):15.
41. Sokol MC, McGuigan KA, Verbrugge RR, et al. Impact of medication adherence on hospitalization risk and healthcare cost. Med Care 2005;43(6):521–30.
42. Rasmussen JN, Chong A, Alter DA. Relationship between adherence to evidence-based pharmacotherapy and long-term mortality after acute myocardial infarction. JAMA 2007;297(2):177–86.
43. Gorard DA. Escalating polypharmacy. QJM 2006;99(11):797–800.
44. Fincke BG, Snyder K, Cantillon C, et al. Three complementary definitions of polypharmacy: methods, application and comparison of findings in a large prescription database. Pharmacoepidemiol Drug Saf 2005;14(2):121–8.
45. Rollason V, Vogt N. Reduction of polypharmacy in the elderly: a systematic review of the role of the pharmacist. Drugs Aging 2003;20(11):817–32.
46. Beers MH, Ouslander JG, Rollingher I, et al. Explicit criteria for determining inappropriate medication use in nursing home residents. UCLA Division of Geriatric Medicine. Arch Intern Med 1991;151(9):1825–32.
47. Naugler CT, Brymer C, Stolee P, et al. Development and validation of an improving prescribing in the elderly tool. Can J Clin Pharmacol 2000;7(2):103–7.
48. Barry PJ, Gallagher P, Ryan C, et al. START (screening tool to alert doctors to the right treatment)–an evidence-based screening tool to detect prescribing omissions in elderly patients. Age Ageing 2007;36(6):632–8.
49. Gallagher P, Ryan C, Byrne S, et al. STOPP (Screening Tool of Older Person's Prescriptions) and START (Screening Tool to Alert doctors to Right Treatment). Consensus validation. Int J Clin Pharmacol Ther 2008;46(2):72–83.
50. McLeod PJ, Huang AR, Tamblyn RM, et al. Defining inappropriate practices in prescribing for elderly people: a national consensus panel. CMAJ 1997;156(3):385–91.
51. Hanlon JT, Schmader KE, Samsa GP, et al. A method for assessing drug therapy appropriateness. J Clin Epidemiol 1992;45(10):1045–51.
52. Klarin I, Wimo A, Fastbom J. The association of inappropriate drug use with hospitalisation and mortality: a population-based study of the very old. Drugs Aging 2005;22(1):69–82.

53. Aparasu RR, Mort JR. Inappropriate prescribing for the elderly: beers criteria-based review. Ann Pharmacother 2000;34(3):338–46.

54. Steinman MA, Landefeld CS, Rosenthal GE, et al. Polypharmacy and prescribing quality in older people. J Am Geriatr Soc 2006;54(10):1516–23.

55. Viktil KK, Blix HS, Reikvam ÅA. The janus face of polypharmacy - overuse versus underuse of medication. Norsk Epidemiologi 2008;18(2):147–52.

56. Hagstrom B, Mattsson B, Wimo A, et al. More illness and less disease? A 20-year perspective on chronic disease and medication. Scand J Public Health 2006;34(6): 584–8.

57. Ananth J, Parameswaran S, Gunatilake S. Side effects of atypical antipsychotic drugs. Curr Pharm Des 2004;10(18):2219–29.

58. McGavock H. Prescription-related illness–a scandalous pandemic. J Eval Clin Pract 2004;10(4):491–7.

59. Chutka DS, Takahashi PY, Hoel RW. Inappropriate medication use in the elderly. Essent Psychopharmacol 2005;6(6):331–40.

60. Ananth J, Parameswaran S, Gunatilake S. Antipsychotic polypharmacy. Curr Pharm Des 2004;10(18):2231–8.

61. Hovstadius B, Astrand B, Petersson G. Dispensed drugs and multiple medications in the Swedish population: an individual-based register study. BMC Clin Pharmacol 2009;9(1):11.

62. Viola R, Csukonyi K, Doro P, et al. Reasons for polypharmacy among psychiatric patients. Pharm World Sci 2004;26(3):143–7.

63. Jyrkka J, Enlund H, Korhonen MJ, et al. Patterns of drug use and factors associated with polypharmacy and excessive polypharmacy in elderly persons: results of the Kuopio 75+ study: a cross-sectional analysis. Drugs Aging 2009;26(6):493–503.

64. Pappa E, Kontodimopoulos N, Papadopoulos AA, et al. Prescribed-drug utilization and polypharmacy in a general population in Greece: association with sociodemo-graphic, health needs, health-services utilization, and lifestyle factors. Eur J Clin Pharmacol 2011;67(2):185–92.

65. Al-Windi A, Elmfeldt D, Svardsudd K. Determinants of drug utilisation in a Swedish municipality. Pharmacoepidemiol Drug Saf 2004;13(2):97–103.

66. Perry BA, Turner LW. A prediction model for polypharmacy: are older, educated women more susceptible to an adverse drug event? J Women Aging 2001;13(4): 39–51.

67. Linjakumpu T. Drug use among the home-dwelling elderly. Trend, polypharmacy, and sedation. Oulu (Finland): University of Oulu; 2003.

68. Odubanjo E, Bennett K, Feely J. Influence of socioeconomic status on the quality of prescribing in the elderly–a population based study. Br J Clin Pharmacol 2004;58(5): 496–502.

69. Hovstadius B, Astrand B, Petersson G. Assessment of regional variation in polyphar-macy. Pharmacoepidemiol Drug Saf 2010;19:375–83.

70. Fastbom J. [Increased consumption of drugs among the elderly results in greater risk of problems]. Lakartidningen 2001;98(14):1674–9 [in Swedish].

71. Queneau P. [Pitfalls of polypharmacy, particularly in the elderly]. Bull Mem Acad R Med Belg 2006;161(6):408–21 [discussion: 422–4] [in French].

72. Chan DC, Hao YT, Wu SC. Characteristics of outpatient prescriptions for frail Taiwanese elders with long-term care needs. Pharmacoepidemiol Drug Saf 2009; 18(4):327–34.

73. Cleland JG, Baksh A, Louis A. Polypharmacy (or polytherapy) in the treatment of heart failure. Heart Fail Monit 2000;1(1):8–13.

74. Bjerrum L. Pharmacoepidemiological studies of polypharmacy: methodological issues, population estimates, and influence of practice patterns. Odense (Denmark): Odense University Denmark; 1998.
75. Hovstadius B, Tågerud S, Petersson G, et al. Prevalence and therapeutic intensity of dispensed drug groups for individuals with multiple medications: a register-based study of 2.2 million individuals. J Pharm Health Serv Res 2010;1:145–55.
76. Bushardt RL, Jones KW. Nine key questions to address polypharmacy in the elderly. JAAPA 2005;18(5):32–7.
77. Frank C, Godwin M, Verma S, et al. What drugs are our frail elderly patients taking? Do drugs they take or fail to take put them at increased risk of interactions and inappropriate medication use? Can Fam Physician 2001;47:1198–204.
78. Nisly NL, Gryzlak BM, Zimmerman MB, et al. Dietary supplement polypharmacy: an unrecognized public health problem? Evid Based Complement Alternat Med 2010; 7(1):107–13.
79. Anthierens S, Tansens A, Petrovic M, et al. Qualitative insights into general practitioners views on polypharmacy. BMC Fam Pract 2010;11:65.
80. Moen J, Norrgård S, Antonov K, et al. GPs' perceptions of multiple-medicine use in older patients. J Eval Clin Pract 2010;16:69–75.
81. Petersen EE, Rasmussen SA, Daniel KL, et al. Prescription medication borrowing and sharing among women of reproductive age. J Womens Health (Larchmt) 2008;17(7): 1073–80.
82. Goldsworthy RC, Schwartz NC, Mayhorn CB. Beyond abuse and exposure: framing the impact of prescription-medication sharing. Am J Public Health 2008; 98(6):1115–21.
83. Grimmsmann T, Himmel W. Polypharmacy in primary care practices: an analysis using a large health insurance database. Pharmacoepidemiol Drug Saf 2009;18(12): 1206–13.
84. Bjerrum L, Sogaard J, Hallas J, et al. Polypharmacy in general practice: differences between practitioners. Br J Gen Pract 1999;49(440):195–8.
85. Gillespie U, Alassaad A, Henrohn D, et al. A comprehensive pharmacist intervention to reduce morbidity in patients 80 years or older: a randomized controlled trial. Arch Intern Med 2009;169(9):894–900.
86. Kragh A. [Two out of three persons living in nursing homes for the elderly are treated with at least ten different drugs. A survey of drug prescriptions in the northeastern part of Skane]. Lakartidningen 2004;101(11):994–6, 999 [in Swedish].
87. Salazar JA, Poon I, Nair M. Clinical consequences of polypharmacy in elderly: expect the unexpected, think the unthinkable. Expert Opin Drug Saf 2007;6(6):695–704.
88. Tinetti ME, Bogardus ST Jr, Agostini JV. Potential pitfalls of disease-specific guidelines for patients with multiple conditions. N Engl J Med 2004;351(27):2870–4.
89. Boyd CM, Darer J, Boult C, et al. Clinical practice guidelines and quality of care for older patients with multiple comorbid diseases: implications for pay for performance. JAMA 2005;294(6):716–24.
90. Rossi MI, Young A, Maher R, et al. Polypharmacy and health beliefs in older outpatients. Am J Geriatr Pharmacother 2007;5(4):317–23.
91. Rochon PA, Gurwitz JH. Optimising drug treatment for elderly people: the prescribing cascade. BMJ 1997;315(7115):1096–9.
92. Walsh EK, Cussen K. "Take ten minutes": a dedicated ten minute medication review reduces polypharmacy in the elderly. Ir Med J 2010;103(8):236–8.
93. Ito H, Koyama A, Higuchi T. Polypharmacy and excessive dosing: psychiatrists' perceptions of antipsychotic drug prescription. Br J Psychiatry 2005;187:243–7.

94. Green JL, Hawley JN, Rask KJ. Is the number of prescribing physicians an independent risk factor for adverse drug events in an elderly outpatient population? Am J Geriatr Pharmacother 2007;5(1):31–9.
95. Little P, Dorward M, Warner G, et al. Importance of patient pressure and perceived pressure and perceived medical need for investigations, referral, and prescribing in primary care: nested observational study. BMJ 2004;328(7437):444.

Polypharmacy, Adverse Drug Reactions, and Geriatric Syndromes

Bhavik M. Shah, PharmD, BCPS*, Emily R. Hajjar, PharmD, BCPS, BCACP, CGP

KEYWORDS

- Polypharmacy • Elderly • Geriatric syndromes
- Adverse drug reactions

The older population, composed of adults aged 65 years or older, is the fastest growing segment of the United States population. The Administration of Aging of the United States Department of Health and Human Services reported that there were approximately 40 million older adults in 2009, an increase of 12.5% from 1999. The Administration projects the greatest increases to the older population to occur over the next two decades as the first baby boomers reach the age of 65 in 2011. By 2030, there will be approximately 72 million older adults.[1] Chronic diseases are prevalent among the older population; about 80% of older adults have at least one chronic condition, and about half have at least two.[2] These chronic conditions, which include heart disease, hypertension, diabetes, arthritis, and cancer, often require multiple medications for optimal management.

Although the use of multiple medications is widely referred to as polypharmacy, no consensus exists on what number should define the term. In the literature, polypharmacy has been arbitrarily defined as taking at least two to nine medications concurrently.[3–7] This definition is controversial because polypharmacy may be appropriate to treat a patient with multiple comorbid conditions. This appropriateness is especially true for disease states such as chronic heart failure and diabetes, which require multiple drug therapies as directed by disease state guidelines. For example, a patient with Class IV New York Heart Association heart failure may be prescribed a loop diuretic, an aldosterone inhibiting diuretic, a β-blocker, an angiotensin-converting enzyme inhibitor, digoxin to treat the heart failure, and other medications for any other comorbid condition. Excessive polypharmacy is another type of polypharmacy that is defined by medication count and generally uses cut points of 10 or more

B. Shah has no relationships to disclose.
E. Hajjar is a consultant for Prime Therapeutics.
Jefferson School of Pharmacy, Thomas Jefferson University, 130 South 9th Street, Suite 1540, Philadelphia, PA 19107, USA
* Corresponding author.
E-mail address: bhavik.shah@jefferson.edu

Clin Geriatr Med 28 (2012) 173–186
doi:10.1016/j.cger.2012.01.002
0749-0690/12/$ – see front matter © 2012 Elsevier Inc. All rights reserved.
geriatric.theclinics.com

medications. This definition is becoming increasingly studied as the population continues to age and use more medications.

Alternately, polypharmacy has also been defined as taking at least one medication that is not clinically indicated. This indication-based definition is argued to be more practical and appropriate because it is independent of the multiple medications necessary to treat the multiple comorbidities elderly patients are likely to have.[7] This definition necessitates a medication review and takes medication appropriateness into account. Those that lack an indication or effectiveness or are determined to be a therapeutic duplication are considered as polypharmacy or unnecessary medications. An example would be a patient started on a proton pump inhibitor while an inpatient for stress ulcer prophylaxis. If the medication is continued on an outpatient basis, this medication would be considered unnecessary because there is no longer an indication for the medication.

EPIDEMIOLOGY
Prevalence of Polypharmacy Defined by Medication Count

Overall medication use has increased recently. According to IMS Health data, the number of prescriptions filled in 2010 was about 4 billion.[8] Although making up about 13% of the US population, older adults filled one-third of all prescriptions and 40% of nonprescription medications.[9] The average older adult filled 31 prescriptions per year in 2009, twice as many as all other age groups combined.[10] Similar disproportionate use has been reported in Canada and the United Kingdom.[11,12]

The prevalence of polypharmacy reported in the literature, ranging from 5% to 78%, varies because of the different definitions used and samples studied.[7] Furthermore, the reported average number of prescriptions taken daily by ambulatory elderly patients ranges between two and nine medications.[13] Polypharmacy is more common in women, and its prevalence increases with advancing age.[7] A large national survey of prescription and nonprescription medication use in ambulatory adults found that 57% of women aged 65 years or older took at least five medications, and 12% took at least 10 medications.[14] A European study of ambulatory older adults reported a similar prevalence rate; 51% of elderly patients took at least six prescription and nonprescription medications per day.[15]

Nobili and colleagues[16] reported the rate of polypharmacy among hospitalized Italian elderly patients of 52% with a mean number of 4.9 medications (N = 1332, mean age 79.4 years) upon admission; the rate of polypharmacy increased to 67% upon discharge with a mean number of 6.0 medications.[16] Schuler and colleagues[17] reported a polypharmacy rate of 58% upon admission in Austrian hospitals, with a mean number of 7.5 medications (N = 543, median age 82 years). In the United States, about half of elderly patients admitted to hospitals take seven or more medications.[18]

A large national study of 13,507 nursing home residents showed a polypharmacy rate of 40%. Polypharmacy was defined as at least nine medications, a higher threshold compared with other studies in ambulatory or hospitalized settings.[19] Data on the prevalence rate in assisted living facilities is more limited. However, one study of 2014 residents, the majority of whom were 85 years or older, in 193 assisted living facilities reported a mean of 5.8 medications.[20]

Prevalence of Polypharmacy Defined as Unnecessary Drug Use

Medication use that is not clinically warranted is another definition of polypharmacy.[7] Lipton and colleagues[21] found that 60% of 236 ambulatory elderly patients aged 65 years or older were taking medications that lacked an indication or were suboptimal. In a study of 196 elderly veteran patients, Steinman and colleagues[22] evaluated unnecessary medications by using the Medication Appropriateness Index (MAI), defined as medications with no indication, lack of effectiveness, or therapeutic duplication. They reported that 57% of patients were taking at least one unnecessary medication. Using the MAI criteria for unnecessary medication, Schmader and colleagues[23] found that a mean number of 0.65 unnecessary medications were taken in a study of 834 frail elderly veterans. Additionally, a study of 384 hospitalized frail elderly veterans found that 44% of patients were discharged with at least one unnecessary medication, as defined by the MAI.[24] A majority of these patients (75%) had at least one unnecessary medication prior to hospital admission. The most common reason was a lack of indication (33%). Hanlon and colleagues[25] reported similar findings; lack of indication was the most common reason for unnecessary medications in a study of 397 hospitalized elderly veterans. Common unnecessary medications include gastrointestinal, central nervous system, and therapeutic nutrient/mineral agents.[24]

Most Common Medications

Kaufman and colleagues[14] reported in 2002 that the most common prescription medications among ambulatory older patients were conjugated estrogens, levothyroxine, hydrochlorothiazide, atorvastatin, and lisinopril. A study of ambulatory Medicare patients revealed that the most common drug classes prescribed in a 1-year period were cardiovascular agents, antibiotics, diuretics, analgesics, antihyperlipidemics, and gastrointestinal agents.[26] This result is to be expected because the drugs reflect the common conditions that occur in community-dwelling elders. The most common nonprescription medications consumed by older adults were analgesics (aspirin, acetaminophen, and ibuprofen), cough and cold medications (diphenhydramine and pseudoephedrine), vitamins and minerals (multivitamins, vitamins E and C, calcium), and herbal products (ginseng, Ginkgo biloba extract).[14] Other nonprescription medications commonly used by elderly patients include antacids and laxatives.[27] A survey of institutionalized older adults found that the most common medications were gastrointestinal agents, central nervous system agents (antidepressants, antipsychotics, antimanics), and analgesics (opioids and nonopioids).[19]

CONSEQUENCES OF POLYPHARMACY

There are many consequences of polypharmacy. Aside from increased direct drug costs, patients are at higher risk for adverse drug reactions, drug interactions, nonadherence, diminished functional status, and various geriatric syndromes.

Adverse Drug Reactions

The number of adverse drug reactions (ADRs) for all age groups has increased over recent years, with an estimated 4.3 million ADR-related health care visits in 2005.[28] Age 65 years or older and polypharmacy were significant risk factors for ADR-related visits. ADRs occur in up to 35% of outpatients and 44% of hospitalized elderly patients and account for approximately 10% of emergency room visits.[29,30] Polypharmacy increases the risk of ADRs from 13% (two medications) to 58% (five drugs).[31] Seven or more medications further increases the risk of ADRs to 82%.[31] The most common drug classes associated with ADRs were cardiovascular drugs, diuretics, anticoagulants, nonsteroidal antiinflammatory drugs, antibiotics, and hypoglycemics.[26,30] These medications are prescribed for common conditions, and providers should be aware of the risks for each medication class.

Drug Interactions

The elderly are at high risk for drug interactions due to polypharmacy, comorbidities, and decreased nutritional status, which may affect the pharmacokinetic and pharmacodynamic properties of medications.[32] Potential drug-drug interactions are common. In a prospective, randomized controlled longitudinal multicenter European study of 1601 community-dwelling elderly adults, 46% of patients had a potential drug-drug interaction.[33] This result is consistent with other studies that report the prevalence of potential drug-drug interactions between 35% and 60% in elderly patients.[29] The risk of drug-drug interactions increases with the number of drugs and can approach 100% with eight or more medications.[34] In elderly patients, drug-drug interactions are a common reason for preventable adverse drug reactions and hospitalizations related to drug toxicity.[26,35]

The prevalence of drug-disease interactions is reported to be 15% to 40% in frail elderly patients.[36,37] The investigators noted the most common interactions were aspirin and peptic ulcer disease, calcium channel blockers and heart failure, and β-blockers and diabetes. The risk of drug-disease interactions has been shown to increase as the number of drugs as well as the number of comorbidities increase.[37] Risk of drug-disease interactions are of concern because few patients suffer from just one chronic condition.

The prevalence rates should be interpreted cautiously, because they may be overestimated due to how interactions and their clinical importance are defined.[32] Additionally, many of the studies evaluated potential interactions, which may not be clinically relevant.[30] Nevertheless, the elderly are at risk for drug interactions. These interactions are significant because they may decrease the efficacy or increase the risk of toxicity of a drug. As a result, the prescriber may change the dose or add more medications, further increasing the risk for other interactions and side effects.

Nonadherence

Complex medication regimens related to polypharmacy can lead to nonadherence in the elderly.[13] Studies in community-dwelling elderly adults have reported medication adherence rates between 43% and 95%.[38] The variability can be attributed to different definitions for adherence, population characteristics, and how adherence was measured. The number of medications has been shown to be a stronger predictor of nonadherence than advancing age, with higher rates of nonadherence as the number of medications increases.[39,40] Nonadherence can lead to serious sequelae including disease progression, treatment failure, hospitalization, and adverse drug events.[40]

Diminished Activities of Daily Living and Instrumental Activities of Daily Living

Polypharmacy has also been associated with functional decline in older patients. In a prospective study of over 600 community-dwelling elderly, increased prescription medication use was associated with decreased physical functioning and decreased ability to carry out instrumental activities of daily living (IADLs) after controlling for age, education, health, number of conditions, and baseline functional status.[41] Another cross-sectional study based on the Women's Health and Aging Study found that the use of five or more medications resulted in diminished ability to perform IADLs, especially being able to shop for personal items (including medications).[42] Yet another study of approximately 300 patients reported that excessive polypharmacy (using >10 drugs) was associated with a decline in the ability to perform IADLs. Only 30% of patients with no polypharmacy were found to have difficulty performing

IADLs, whereas 74% of those with excessive polypharmacy were found to have difficulty with IADLs.[43] Higher medication use has also been positively associated with functional decline in patients who have suffered a fall in the previous year.[44] Although medication may be used to preserve some functional capacity, providers should be aware of the association between polypharmacy and functional decline.

Increased Health Service Utilization and Resources

The use of multiple medications leads to increased costs for both the patient and the health system as a whole. Whereas the proper use of medications may lead to decreased hospital and emergency room admissions, the use of inappropriate medications may not only increase patients' drug costs but cause them to use more health care services. A retrospective population study in Ireland concluded that approximately 9% of the total drug-related expenditures were on potentially inappropriate medications.[45] Consequences of polypharmacy can also lead to an increase in health resources as well. A retrospective cohort study of elderly Japanese patients reported that patients with polypharmacy were at risk of having a potentially inappropriate medication, which then increased the risk for hospitalization and outpatient visits and resulted in a 33% increase in medical costs.[46]

Increased Risk of Geriatric Syndromes

Cognitive impairments

Cognitive impairment, which includes delirium and dementia, occurs commonly in the elderly. In a review of 42 cohorts of medical inpatients composed of mostly older adults, the rate of delirium ranged from 11% to 42%.[47] Whereas the cause of delirium is multifactorial, drugs are a common risk factor and may be the precipitating cause in 12% to 39% of cases.[48] Inouye and Charpentier[49] reported that the number of medications (four or more) added the day before a delirium episode was a risk factor for delirium. Another study of 156 hospitalized older adults found that the number of medications was an independent risk factor for delirium.[50] The most common drugs associated with delirium are opioids, benzodiazepines, and anticholinergics. Similarly, drug classes that can exacerbate dementia are benzodiazepines, anticonvulsants, and anticholinergic drugs such as tricyclic antidepressants.[51]

Cognitive impairment measured by the Mini-Mental State Examination (MMSE) has also been found to be negatively associated with polypharmacy. A cohort study of 294 Finnish elders reported that those with polypharmacy were found to have a decrease of 1.36 points in their MMSE scores. Twenty-two percent of patients with no polypharmacy were found to have impaired cognition as opposed to 33% and 54% with polypharmacy and excessive polypharmacy, respectively.[43]

Falls

Falls are an especially concerning problem in the elderly, causing increased morbidity and mortality. Unfortunately, many medications are known to increase the risk of falls. A cross-sectional study in older outpatients found that the number of prescribed medications was significantly associated with the risk of falls.[52] Another study evaluating risk factors for those who have not fallen compared with those who have fallen once and those who have experienced multiple falls found that the number of medications was associated with an increased risk of falls.[53] In the Longitudinal Aging Study Amsterdam, it was found that use of four or more medications was associated with increased risk of falling as well as increased risk of recurrent falls.[54] Other studies have shown there is an increased risk of falls from polypharmacy for both hospital and nursing home populations.[55]

Table 1
Drug regimen review to reduce polypharmacy

Author and Year	Setting	N	Intervention	Results
Muir et al, 2004[63]	General medicine inpatient service in Veterans Affairs medical center	836	Medication grid provided to admitting residents that included all medications and administration times over 1 week.	Number of medications reduced in intervention group (−0.92) compared with control (+1.65), as well as the mean number of doses (−2.47 vs +3.83, respectively). ($P<.001$ for both).
Zarowitz et al, 2005[64]	Outpatient, managed care	6693 (first intervention) 6039 (second intervention)	Clinical pharmacists reviewed drug regimens, educated physicians and patients on polypharmacy, and worked with physicians to reduce polypharmacy.	The rate of polypharmacy reduced by 67.5% after first intervention, from 29.01 to 9.43 events/1000 patients. After the second intervention, the polypharmacy rate was reduced by 39%, from 27.99 to 17.07 events/1000 patients.
Schamder et al, 2004[23]	Inpatient and outpatient frail elderly veterans	834	Inpatient and outpatient geriatric evaluation and management consisting of geriatrician, nurse, social worker, and pharmacist.	Geriatric evaluation and management reduced the number of unnecessary and inappropriate drugs in inpatients ($P<.05$), but not in outpatients.
Hanlon et al, 1996[65]	Outpatient veterans	208	Clinical pharmacist reviewed regimens and communicated recommendations in writing and verbally to primary physician.	Using the Medication Appropriateness Index, inappropriate prescribing significantly decreased in the intervention group compared with the control at 3 months (decrease of 24% versus 6%, respectively, $P = .0006$). This benefit was sustained at 12 months (decrease 28% vs 5%, $P = .002$). This result included lower rates of unnecessary medications in the intervention group based on descriptive data.

Galt, 1998[66]	Outpatient veterans	336	Pharmacist pharmacotherapy consult.	Reduced average number of prescriptions per patient (2.4).
Fillit et al, 1999[67]	Outpatient Medicare beneficiaries	5737 surveyed, 2615 (46%) responded, 1087 went to physician	Elderly Medicare beneficiaries at risk for polypharmacy were sent letters by managed care organization encouraging them to meet with their primary physicians for medication review. Physicians provided with guidelines on polypharmacy.	Of the 1087 patients who scheduled a medication review, 20% reported having a medication discontinued.
Fick et al, 2004[68]	Medicare and Choice southeastern managed care organization primary care physicians and patients	355 physicians	Physicians were mailed a listing of patients who were taking potentially inappropriate medications, as defined by the Beer's criteria, as well as alternative recommendations provided by multiple independent pharmacists and geriatricians.	12.5% of potentially inappropriate medications were discontinued. The most common discontinued medications were antihistamines, analgesics, and muscle relaxants.

Use of certain medications is also of concern when considering risk factors for falls in older adults. Psychotropic and cardiovascular medications are of particular concern because of their association with increased risk of falls.[56,57] In a study of over 300 community-dwelling male veterans, the use of a psychotropic medication was associated with an increased risk of falls (odds ratio [OR] 1.54; 95% confidence interval [CI] 1.07–2.22). The use of two or more psychotropic medications further increased the risk of falls in this population (OR 2.37; 95% CI 1.14–4.94).[58] A population-based cohort study of over 2000 Swedish patients evaluated the prevalence of polypharmacy before and after reported hip fracture. Interestingly, the use of five or more medications was seen in 48% percent of the population before they fractured a hip compared with 88% after the hip fracture. The proportion of patients taking 10 or more medication as well as those taking three or more psychotropic medication also increased after hip fracture.[59] This trend of increasing polypharmacy after a traumatic event such as a hip fracture is of concern because the use of multiple medications puts the patient at risk for the original event. The risk of further events is likely to increase, and providers should be aware of this trend and the risk that each type of medication carries with regard to falls.

Urinary incontinence

Urinary incontinence is yet another problem that commonly affects older adults, and the use of multiple medications can exacerbate the problem. A retrospective study of 128 patients found that approximately 60% of patients with urinary incontinence were on at least four medications.[60] A cross-sectional study found that medications that cause polyuria, decreased sensory input, and decreased bladder contractility were associated with the patient's self-reported urinary incontinence.[61]

Nutrition

Polypharmacy also puts elders at increased risk of poor nutritional status. A survey conducted in community-dwelling elders aged 65 and older reported that polypharmacy was associated with poorer nutritional status. Higher medication use was associated with a decreased intake of soluble and nonsoluble fiber, fat-soluble vitamins, B vitamins, and minerals and an increased intake of cholesterol, glucose, and sodium.[62] A prospective cohort study found that nutritional assessment measured by the mini-nutritional assessment–short version was also negatively impacted by polypharmacy. Only 10% of patients with no polypharmacy were found to be either malnourished or at risk of malnourishment as compared with 50% in those with excessive polypharmacy.[43]

CLINICAL APPROACH TO IMPROVING POLYPHARMACY
Drug Regimen Review

Several studies support reviewing drug regimens to reduce polypharmacy.[23,63–68] These studies have been conducted in inpatient and ambulatory settings, with regimens reviewed by physicians, pharmacists, and/or managed care organizations. The studies are summarized in **Table 1**.

Principles for Optimizing Drug Use in the Elderly

Extensive medication histories should be obtained at the initial visit and updated with each subsequent encounter. Medication histories should include both prescription and nonprescription medications and any other health-related food or drink the patient is consuming. Patients and/or their caregivers should be encouraged to bring in all prescription and over-the-counter (OTC) products with them to each health care visit. If the patient cannot bring in the actual products, an updated list of all medications should be kept with the patient to give to all providers so health records can be kept as up-to-date as possible. Both primary care and specialist providers need to have inclusive lists as to not create polypharmacy because of incomplete health care related data. Additional questioning is most likely needed to ascertain all of the OTC products that a patient takes. Items such as vitamins, supplements, and OTC items such as antacids may be inadvertently left off medication lists or not be included with other medications, because patients often perceive these to be without risk or unimportant for the health care provider to know about. Informing patients or caregivers of drug interactions with nonprescription agents may be one way to stress the importance of providing a comprehensive list of medications to all providers.

Once a complete medication list has been obtained, the provider can then determine if a medication is warranted and if the benefits outweigh the risks for that drug. All medications should have an indication, and if they do not, an evaluation is needed to see if the medication is necessary. Discontinuation of unnecessary medications is reasonable for most drugs, but some may need to be tapered off to prevent any adverse drug withdrawal events. It is also important to determine if a new medication is being used to treat the side effects of another medication. Although sometimes a prescribing cascade is necessary (eg, potassium supplementation in a patient receiving a diuretic), many times it adds an unnecessary burden to the patient's already complicated medication regimen. Existing therapies should also be evaluated to determine if they need to be continued or if optimization could occur. As patients age and their health status changes, medications may become ineffective, more harmful, or require dosage changes to prevent ADRs from occurring. Nonpharmacologic therapy, such as diet and exercise, should be considered whenever possible. If a medication is determined to be necessary, health care providers need to consider the medication's pharmacokinetic and pharmacodynamic properties, side effect profile, and current hepatic and renal function for accurate dosing. Medication cost, patient preference, and potential for drug-drug and drug-disease interactions should also be considered in prescribing. Reasonable therapeutic goals and monitoring parameters will help guide therapy to prevent unwanted side effects. It is also wise for health care providers to create their own personal formularies where they become very familiar with prescribing a few drugs. Simplifying medication regimens as well as educating patients regarding medications can improve adherence.[69] Adherence may also be improved with the use of generic medications whenever possible, pill boxes and other adherence tools, and educating caregivers.

Two techniques, often referred to as SAIL and TIDE, are helpful in remembering ways to reduce polypharmacy.[9] Summarized in **Table 2**, they refer to the following:

- **S**imple: Keep the regimen as simple as possible. Use medications that can be dosed once or twice a day. Use a medication that can treat multiple indications. When drug therapy has been titrated to ideal doses, try to combine medications into single pills to reduce pill burden.
- **A**dverse effects: Know the potential adverse effects of medications. Choose medications that have broad therapeutic indices when possible. Identify medications that are treating adverse effects of other medications. Discontinue the drug that is causing the adverse effect, if possible.
- **I**ndication: Ensure each medication has an indication and a defined, realistic therapeutic goal.

Table 2
SAIL and TIDE techniques to reduce polypharmacy[9]

Technique	Description
SAIL	
Simplify	Simplify drug regimens to reduce pill burden. Use medications that can be dosed once or twice daily. Use medications that can treat multiple conditions.
Adverse effects	Be familiar with adverse effects of medications. Choose medications that have broad therapeutic indices when possible. Discontinue a medication that is causing an adverse effect when possible.
Indication	Ensure each medication has an indication and a defined, realistic therapeutic goal.
List	List the name and dose of each medication in the chart and share it with the patient and/or caregiver.
TIDE	
Time	Allow sufficient time to address and discuss medication issues during each encounter.
Individualize	Apply pharmacokinetic and pharmacodynamic principles to individualize medication regimens. Consider dose adjustments for renal and/or hepatic impairment. Start medications at lower doses than usual and titrate slowly.
Drug interactions	Consider potential drug-drug and drug-disease interactions. Avoid potentially dangerous interactions, such as those that can increase the risk for torsades de pointes.
Educate	Educate the patient and caregiver regarding pharmacologic and nonpharmacologic treatments. Discuss expected medication effects, potential adverse effects, and monitoring parameters.

- List: Write down the name and dose of each medication in the chart and share it with the patient.
- Time: Allow sufficient time to address and discuss medication issues.
- Individualize: Apply pharmacokinetic and pharmacodynamic principles to individual patients to select the most appropriate medication and dose. Consider dose adjustments for the patient's renal or hepatic function. Medications should start at lower than usual doses and be titrated slowly, often referred to as "start low, go slow."
- Drug-drug and drug-disease interactions: Consider potential drug-drug and drug-disease interactions, and avoid potentially dangerous interactions such as those leading to torsades de pointes.
- Educate: Educate the patient and caregiver regarding pharmacologic and nonpharmacologic treatments. Discuss expected medication effects, potential adverse effects, and drug-drug interactions and monitoring parameters.

SUMMARY

The elderly are at risk for polypharmacy, which is associated with significant consequences such as adverse effects, medication nonadherence, drug-drug and drug-disease interactions, and increased risk of geriatric syndromes. Providers should evaluate all existing medications at each patient visit for appropriateness and weigh the risks and benefits of starting new medications to minimize polypharmacy.

REFERENCES

1. Administration on Aging of the United State Department of Health and Human Services. A profile of older Americans: 2010. Available at: http://www.aoa.gov/aoaroot/aging_statistics/Profile/2010/docs/2010profile.pdf. Updated February 25, 2011. Accessed August 10, 2011.
2. Centers for Disease Control and Prevention. Public health and aging: trends in aging — United States and worldwide. MMWR Morb Mortal Wkly Rep 2003;52:101–10.
3. Stewart RB, Cooper JW. Polypharmacy in the aged. Practical solutions. Drugs Aging 1994;4:449–61.
4. Bikowski R, Ripsin C, Lorraine V. Physician-patient congruence regarding medication regimens. J Am Geriatr Soc 2001;49:1353–7.
5. Joorgensen T, Johansson S, Kennerfalk A, et al. Prescription drug use, diagnoses, and healthcare utilization among the elderly. Ann Pharmacother 2001;35:1004–9.
6. Linjakumpu T, Hartkainen S, Klaukka T, et al. Use of medications and polypharmacy are increasing among the elderly. J Clin Epidemiol 2002;55:809–17.
7. Fulton MM, Allen ER. Polypharmacy in the elderly: a literature review. J Am Acad Nurse Pract 2005;17:123–32.
8. Top-line Market Data. IMS Health Web site. Available at: http://www.imshealth.com/deployedfiles/ims/Global/Content/Corporate/Press%20Room/Top-line%20Market%20Data/2010%20Top-line%20Market%20Data/2010_Top_Therapeutic_Classes_by_RX.pdf. Accessed August 18, 2011.
9. Werder SF, Preskorn SH. Managing polypharmacy: walking a fine line between help and harm. Current Psychiatry Online. 2003;2. Available at: http://www.jfponline.com/Pages.asp?AID=601. Accessed August 20, 2011.
10. United States prescription drugs. Kaiser Family Health Foundation. Available at: http://www.statehealthfacts.org/profileind.jsp?sub=66&rgn=1&cat=5. Accessed August 20, 2011.
11. Barat I, Andreasen F, Damsgaard EM. The consumption of drugs by 75-year-old individuals living in their own homes. Eur J Clin Pharmacol 2000;56:501–9.
12. Kennerfalk A, Ruigomez A, Wallander MA, et al. Geriatric drug therapy and healthcare utilization in the United Kingdom. Ann Pharmacother 2002;36:797–803.
13. Hajjar ER, Cafiero AC, Hanlon JT. Polypharmacy in elderly patients. Am J Geriatr Pharmacother 2007;5:345–51.
14. Kaufman D, Kelly J, Rosenberg L, et al. Recent patterns of medication use in the ambulatory adult population of the United States: The Slone survey. JAMA 2002;287:337–44.
15. Fialova D, Topinkova E, Gamrassi G, et al. Potentially inappropriate medication use among elderly home care patients in Europe. JAMA 2005;293:1348–58.
16. Nobili A, Licata G, Salerno F, et al. Polypharmacy, length of hospital stay, and in-hospital mortality among elderly patients in internal medicine wards. The REPOSI study. Eur J Clin Pharmacol 2011;67:507–19.
17. Schuler J, Dückelmann C, Beindl W, et al. Polypharmacy and inappropriate prescribing in elderly internal-medicine patients in Austria. Wien Klin Wochenschr 2008;120:733–41.
18. Flaherty JH, Perry HM 3rd, Lynchard GS, et al. Polypharmacy and hospitalization among older home care patients. J Gerontol A Biol Sci Med Sci 2000;55:554–9.
19. Dwyer LL, Han B, Woodwell DA, et al. Polypharmacy in nursing home residents in the United States: results of the 2004 National Nursing Home Survey. Am J Geriatr Pharmacother 2010;8:63–72.

20. Sloane PD, Zimmerman S, Brown LC, et al. Inappropriate medication prescribing in residential care/assisted living facilities. J Am Geriatr Soc 2002;50:1001–11.
21. Lipton HL, Bero LA, Bird JA, et al. The impact of clinical pharmacists' consultations on physicians' geriatric drug prescribing. A randomized controlled trial. Med Care 1992; 30:646–58.
22. Steinman MA, Landerfeld CS, Rosenthal GE, et al. Polypharmacy and prescribing quality in older people. J Am Geriatr Soc 2006;54:1516–23.
23. Schmader KE, Hanlon JT, Pieper CF, et al. Effects of geriatric evaluation and management on adverse reactions and suboptimal prescribing in the frail elderly. Am J Med 2004;116:394–401.
24. Hajjar ER, Hanlon JT, Sloane RJ, et al. Unnecessary drug use in frail older people at hospital discharge. J Am Geriatr Soc 2005;53:1518–23.
25. Hanlon JT, Artz MB, Pieper CF, et al. Inappropriate medication use among frail elderly inpatients. Ann Pharmacother 2004;38:9–14.
26. Gurwitz JH, Field TS, Harrold LR, et al. Incidence and preventability of adverse drug events among older persons in the ambulatory setting. JAMA 2003;289:1107–16.
27. Stoehr GP, Ganguli M, Seaberg EC, et al. Over-the-counter medication use in an older rural community: the MoVIES project. J Am Geriatr Soc 1997;45:158–65.
28. Bourgeois FT, Shannon MW, Valim C, et al. Adverse drug events in the outpatient setting: an 11-year national analysis. Pharmacoepidemiol Drug Saf 2010;19:901–10.
29. Rollason V, Vogt N. Reduction of polypharmacy in the elderly. A systematic review of the role of the pharmacist. Drugs Aging 2003;20:817–32.
30. Hohl CM, Dankoff J, Colacone A, et al. Polypharmacy, adverse drug-related events, and potential adverse drug interactions in elderly patients presenting to an emergency department. Ann Emerg Med 2001;38:666–71.
31. Prybys K, Melville K, Hanna J, et al. Polypharmacy in the elderly: Clinical challenges in emergency practice: Part 1: Overview, etiology, and drug interactions. Emerg Med Rep 2002;23:145–53.
32. Mallet L, Spinewine A, Huang A. The challenge of managing drug interactions in elderly people. Lancet 2007;370:185–91.
33. Bjorkman IK, Fastbom J, Schmidt IK, et al. Drug-drug interactions in the elderly. Ann Pharmacother 2002;36:1675–81
34. Sloan RW. Drug interactions. Am Fam Physician 1983;27:229–38.
35. Juurlink DN, Mamdani M, Kopp A, et al. Drug-drug interactions among elderly patients hospitalized for drug toxicity. JAMA 2003;289:1652–8.
36. Lindblad CI, Hanlon JT, Gross CR, et al. Clinically important drug-disease interactions and their prevalence in older adults. Clin Ther 2006;28:1133–43.
37. Lindblad CI, Artz MB, Pieper CF, et al. Potential drug-disease interactions in frail, hospitalized elderly veterans. Ann Pharmacother 2005;39:412–7.
38. Vik SA, Maxwell CJ, Hogan DB. Measurement, correlates, and health outcomes of medication adherence among seniors. Ann Pharmacother 2004;38:303–12.
39. Colley CA, Lucas LM. Polypharmacy: the cure becomes the disease. J Gen Int Med 1993;8:278–83.
40. Salazar JA, Poon I, Nair M. Clinical consequences of polypharmacy in the elderly: expect the unexpected, think the unthinkable. Expert Opin Drug Saf 2007;6:695–704.
41. Magaziner J, Cadigan DA, Fedder DO, et al. Medication use and functional decline among community-dwelling older women. J Aging Health 1989;1:470–84.
42. Crenstil V, Ricks MO, Xue QL, et al. A pharmacoepidemiologic study of community-dwelling, disabled older women: factors associated with medication use. Am J Geriatr Pharmacother 2010;8:215–24.

43. Jyrkka J, Enlund H, Lavikainen P, et al. Association of polypharmacy with nutritional status, functional ability and cognitive capacity over a three-year period in an elderly population. Pharmacoepidemiol Drug Saf 2010;20:514–22.
44. Stel VS, Smit JH, Plujim SM, et al. Consequences of falling in older men and women and risk factors for health service use and functional decline. Age Aging 2004;33:58–65.
45. Cahir C, Fahey T, Teeling M, et al. Potentially inappropriate prescribing and cost outcomes for older people: a national population study. Br J Clin Pharmacol 2010; 69:543–52.
46. Akazawa M, Imai H, Igarashi A, et al. Potentially inappropriate medication use in elderly Japanese patients. Am J Geriatr Pharmacother 2010;8:146–60.
47. Siddiqi N, Horne AO, Holmes JD. Occurrence and outcome of delirium in medical in-patients: a systematic literature review. Age Ageing 2006;35:350–64.
48. Alagiakrishnan K, Wiens CA. An approach to drug-induced delirium in the elderly. Postgrad Med J 2004;80:388–93.
49. Inouye SK, Charpentier PA. Precipitating factors for delirium in hospitalized elderly persons: predictive model and interrelationship with baseline vulnerability. JAMA 1996;275:852–7.
50. Martin NJ, Stones MJ, Young JE, et al. Development of delirium: a prospective cohort study in a community hospital. Int Psychogeriatr 2000;12:117–27.
51. Hayes BD, Klein-Schwartz W, Barrueto F Jr. Polypharmacy and the geriatric patient. Clin Geriatr Med 2007;23:371–90.
52. Kojima T, Akishita M, Nakamura T, et al. Association of polypharmacy with fall risk among geriatric outpatients. Geriatr Gerontol Int 2011;11:438–44.
53. Fletcher PC, Berg K, Dalby DM, et al. Risk factors for falling among community-based seniors. J Patient Saf 2009;5:61–6.
54. Tromp AM, Plujim SM, Smit JH, et al. Fall-risk screening test: a positive study of predictors for falls in community-dwelling elderly. J Clin Epidemiol 2001;54:837–44.
55. Boyle N, Naganathan V, Cumming RG. Medication and falls: risk and optimization. Clin Geriatr Med 2010;26:583–605.
56. Leipzig RM, Cumming RG, Tinetti ME. Drugs and falls in older people: a systematic review and meta-analysis: I. Psychotropic drugs. J Am Geriatr Soc 1999;47:30–9.
57. Leipzig RM, Cumming RG, Tinetti ME. Drugs and falls in older people: a systematic review and meta-analysis: II. Cardiac and analgesic drugs. J Am Geriatri Soc 1999; 47:40–50.
58. Weiner DK, Hanlon JT, Studenski SA. Effects of central nervous system polypharmacy on falls liability in community-dwelling elderly. Gerontol 1998;44:217–21.
59. Kragh A, Elmstahl S, Atroshi I. Older adults medication use 6 months before and after hip fracture: A population-based cohort study. J Am Geriatr Soc 2011;58:863–8.
60. Gormely EA, Griffiths DJ, McCracken PN, et al. Polypharmacy and its effect of urinary incontinence in a geriatric population. Br J Urol 1993;71:265–9.
61. Ruby CM, Hanlon JT, Fillenbaum GG, et al. Medication use and control of urination among community-dwelling older adults. J Aging Health 2005;17:661–74.
62. Heuberger RA, Caudell K. Polypharmacy and nutritional status in older adults. Drugs Aging 2011;28:315–23.
63. Muir AJ, Sanders LL, Wilkinson WE, et al. Reducing medication regimen complexity. A controlled trial. J Gen Intern Med 2004;16:77–82.
64. Zarowitz BJ, Stebelsky LA, Muma BK, et al. Reduction of high-risk polypharmacy drug combinations in patients in a managed care setting. Pharmacotherapy 2005;25: 1636–45.

65. Hanlon JT, Weinberger M, Samsa GP, et al. A randomized, controlled trial of a clinical pharmacist intervention to improve inappropriate prescribing in elderly outpatients with polypharmacy. Am J Med 1996;100:428–37.

66. Galt KA. Cost avoidance, acceptance, and outcomes associated with a pharmacotherapy consult clinic in a Veterans Affairs Medical Center. Pharmacotherapy 1998; 18:1103–11.

67. Fillit HM, Futterman R, Orland BI, et al. Polypharmacy management in Medicare managed care: changes in prescribing by primary care physicians resulting from a program promoting medication reviews. Am J Manag Care 1999;5:587–94.

68. Fick DM, Maclean JR, Rodriguez NA, et al. A randomized study to decrease the use of potentially inappropriate medications among community-dwelling older adults in a southeastern managed care organization. Am J Manag Care 2004;10:761–8.

69. Schrader SL, Dressing B, Blue R, et al. The medication reduction project: combating polypharmacy in South Dakota elders through community-based interventions. S D J Med 1996;49:441–8.

Clinical Practice Guidelines for Chronic Diseases—Understanding and Managing Their Contribution to Polypharmacy

Ravi P. Ruberu, MB, BS, PhD[a], Stephen P. Fitzgerald, MB, BS, FRACP[b],*

KEYWORDS
- Polypharmacy • Mini polypharmacy
- Hyperpharmacotherapy therapies • Pharmacokinetics
- Pharmacodynamics • Guidelines • Medication

The practice of medicine is strongly influenced by the mathematical interpretation of medical trials. These generally involve randomizing patients to different interventions, analyzing the outcomes, and then choosing the better interventions. There is little doubt that this empiricism has helped the medical profession discard therapies that, although theoretically sound, in fact result in no benefit, or even harm.[1] Also, incremental gains accumulating over time have resulted in improved outcomes in many conditions. Such progress is often summarized in treatment guidelines which, although not dogmatic, set out general standards of care. The management of conditions may then be assessed according to these guidelines.[2–5]

Many individuals, however, especially older people, may have more than one medical condition and are therefore candidates for multiple guideline-supported therapies.[6] All of these therapies are complicated by risk, cost, and inconvenience. The coexistence of multiple therapies is known as polypharmacy, and empirical trials of this entity have demonstrated the significant risks it presents.[5,7] There thus arises the paradox that the following of clinical guidelines so as to benefit individual conditions, when applied repetitively, may result in the emergence of an entity with

Neither author has any commercial or financial disclosures to make.
[a] Department of Geriatric and Rehabilitation Medicine, Royal Adelaide Hospital, Adelaide, SA 5000, Australia
[b] Department of Internal Medicine, Royal Adelaide Hospital, Adelaide, SA 5000, Australia
* Corresponding author.
E-mail address: Stephen.Fitzgerald@health.sa.gov.au

Clin Geriatr Med 28 (2012) 187–198
doi:10.1016/j.cger.2012.01.003   geriatric.theclinics.com
0749-0690/12/$ – see front matter Crown Copyright © 2012 Published by Elsevier Inc. All rights reserved.

significant capacity to cause harm. Medical practitioners who recognize that they treat patients as distinct from individual diseases thus may face a dilemma.[8]

DEFINITIONS AND EPIDEMIOLOGY OF POLYPHARMACY

There are multiple definitions used in literature to describe polypharmacy. Polypharmacy is usually described numerically as five or more prescribed medications at any given time.[9–11] Nevertheless, the European project AgeD in HOme Care (ADHOC) used a number of nine or more medications as a defining figure,[12,13] and there are also qualitative definitions described by various investigators depending on literature that is reviewed. In an attempt to simplify these multiple definitions, Bushardt and colleagues[14] have suggested a change of terminology to reduce ambiguity with terms such as *hyperpharmacotherapy* and *multiple medications*. However, this terminology seems not to have been taken up into the medical vocabulary.

PROBLEM OF POLYPHARMACY

Diseases of chronic nature are cumulative with age, thus raising the number of medications prescribed. Use of multiple medications in the elderly is described in a wide variety of countries that span the globe.[15–20] The advancement of medical science has had minimal impact on reducing the number of medications elderly people are taking, and this trend of polypharmacy has grown over the years.[21]

Prescribing to the elderly has been raised as a complex matter by several investigators with particular attention to medication errors, adverse effects, underutilization, and overutilization.[16,22–24] Furthermore, increasing the number of medications has been shown to correlate well with increasing adverse effects.[25] Beers[26] has developed a set of criteria highlighting drug use by the elderly that has the potential to cause adverse effects. Literature relating to such potentially inappropriate medication (PIM) varies widely between countries. In Europe, North America, and Canada, reported rates vary from 14% to 66%.[27–31] Following several updates since its initial use in residential care patients, the usage of Beers criteria has been extended in to the general community. This usage has occurred in the context of current clinical evidence and knowledge of pharmacokinetics and dynamics.[32] Using Beers criteria and similar approaches, PIM has been studied in multiple communities, showing that its prevalence increases with age and comorbidities as well as with hospital admission; there is also evidence of an increase in mortality and morbidity as a direct result of PIM.[31,33,34] Although PIM can be avoided and has been shown to be declining in the United Kingdom, in certain parts of France and North America it still remains a major problem.[16,35]

Medication regimen complexity index is a validated tool in several communities where it has been used to quantify drug regimen complexities.[36–39] Acurcio Fde and colleagues[40] showed that lower socioeconomic status is a risk factor for increased drug regimen complexity leading to medication errors and noncompliance in the Brazilian community.

Briesacher and colleagues[41] have shown that up to one-third of their study population were noncompliant because of the cost of medications. There have also been reports suggesting that both the burden on the caregiver and the total pill burden are contributory factors to noncompliance.[42,43]

BURDEN OF MULTIPLE ILLNESSES

The population of disabled elderly individuals is sharply rising in many parts of the world. A 300% rise in disabled elderly patients in North America by 2050 has been projected.[44] Currently, an adult over the age of 60 years in North America has on average 2.2 major chronic diseases.[45] Similar trends are noted in the countries of the European Union.[46] According to the Australian Bureau of Statistics, in 2005, 100% of those who were over the age of 65 years claimed they had at least one chronic disease, and 56% reported some form of disability limiting their activities of daily life.[47] These figures are likely to rise with the projected expansion of the elderly population. With the oldest baby boomers reaching 65 years of age in 2011, we are likely to see a disproportionate rise in the elderly with multiple comorbidities on multiple medications.[48]

COST TO THE HEALTH CARE SYSTEMS

With a rapidly increasing number of elderly people, each and every country affected will have to face the challenge of increasing cost of the health care system. These increases not only are due to medication-related issues such as dangerous drug interactions, PIM, and noncompliance but also to the increasing demand for services, which would also substantially increase the financial burden to the community.[33,49]

In response to these pressures, home health care was designed to improve patient care in a cost-effective manner. There is no doubt that this type of care has had made a positive impact over the past few decades. In 1996, the cost of home health care for those who were over 60 years of age in North America reached $27.2 billion. Sixty percent of this cost was paid by Medicare.[50] Out-of-pocket health care cost has increased 104% in this population from $2164 in 1998 to $3748 in 2002.[45] Over 4 years, individuals with two, three, and four chronic medical conditions have had a cost increase in health care of 41%, 85%, and 100%, respectively. These cost increases may have been greater but for the fact of their occurrence in the context of a low-income elderly population with less ability to increase demand as compared with a younger population. Although rather grim projections of increasing health care cost in countries with aging populations have started policy makers thinking of the future, some claim that the projected outcome so far described may not necessarily be true. Using gross domestic product as the denominator, Coory[51] points out several analyses that have shown a better outcome for the future from a financial standpoint. Proponents of this argument state that people will live an increasing period of their lives relatively healthy, requiring less health care expenditure, and the short duration of late diseases of acute nature would cost less because such conditions are more likely to be fatal.[52] However, this argument does not seem to take into account those conditions that are chronic and debilitating and have a higher prevalence in the elderly such as dementing illnesses and cardiac, renal, and pulmonary diseases.

There is a paucity of literature regarding cost burden in relation to iatrogenic diseases in the elderly. In a population-based review of 15,000 patients in North America involving the states of Utah and Colorado, Thomas and Brennan[53] showed that patients aged 65 years or more encounter more preventable adverse events than those who are younger. These events included adverse drug events, falls, and adverse events related to medical procedures.[53] Several other investigators have shown similar findings. Furthermore, on account of increased procedural interventions and hospitalization, a significant increase in nosocomial infections has been also highlighted.[54,55] The prevalence of these adverse outcomes is likely to be similar throughout the world where population demographics and complexity of disease burden share similarities.

Factors governing the use of multiple medications are not limited to aging and chronic diseases but include rather obscure elements such as individual financial burden and race, as well as health-related beliefs.[56] Aggressive marketing campaigns using a wide variety of media including the Internet have reached an unprecedented number of people. Sales of over-the-counter and lifestyle medications, well-known causes of adverse drug interactions and misuse, have grown.[57] With rising consumerism in medicine, Walley[58] points out the increased responsibility that the elderly may have to take in the future. Whereas informed consumerism seems intuitively a helpful safeguarding mechanism, it will no doubt present challenges to health professionals.

The substrate for polypharmacy is thus the increasing population of older patients with multiple illnesses all potentially treated by multiple drugs and procedures. The rationale for all these treatments comes from the analysis of trials and is therefore evidence-based. This rationale is amplified, if not "tainted," by industry and professional imperatives.[59] On the other hand, there are fewer studies, mostly qualitative, concerning the risks of polypharmacy, and no associated commercial champions for decreasing therapy. Potential commercial backers of reduced polypharmacy would include government and other payers.

Although the application of trial data and guideline therapies is rational, there is on deeper thought room for negotiation and individualization of therapy. There are confounding factors and biases that may invalidate such therapies in different circumstances. Scott and Guyatt,[59] stressing the need to avoid both under- and over-treatment of older patients, summarized many confounding and modulating factors that are potential considerations in the extrapolation of trial data to older persons. In particular they focussed on the issues of study design and quality of the evidence, choice of outcome measures, missing outcome data, assessment of potential harm, quantifying treatment effects in individual patients (and adjusting these for effect modifiers and reduced life expectancy), eliciting patient values and preferences, prioritizing therapeutic goals and selection of treatments, and assisting patients in adhering to agreed therapeutic regimens. Awareness of these factors gives a rational basis for the understanding that guidelines are never absolute and that their application to individual patients should rarely be automatic. Scott and Guyatt quote Sackett and colleagues[60] and reiterate the importance of clinical judgement, expertise, and so forth in the practice of evidence-based-medicine. Unfortunately these qualities have been difficult to define and quantify.[60]

Perhaps even more fundamental than these considerations, however, is the appreciation of how marginal a therapy can be in terms of benefit to be regarded as acceptable. Treatment effects are modest. Often many (eg, 50–100) patients need to be treated so that one might benefit. It is an arbitrary judgement as to when this ratio becomes acceptable. Often the ratio is deemed acceptable on the basis of it being similar to the ratio of other treatments, which in turn were justified without specific criteria. The authors have shown that when patients are informed as to the absolute benefits and risks of commonly accepted therapies, they display a range of consequent judgements as to the validity of treatment. In general, in comparison with patients, the medical profession values these same therapies more.[61]

IS POLYPHARMACY ALWAYS BAD?

As discussed previously, polypharmacy has well-described problems and risks. Nevertheless, many patients do tolerate polypharmacy and can manage the adherence issues themselves or with support. It has been argued that, in psychiatry, modern drug development—in other words the designing of drugs with specific, narrow effects so as to maximize tolerability and efficacy—simultaneously creates a need for polypharmacy.[62]

ANALYZING EVIDENCE-BASED MEDICINE IN THE CONTEXT OF MULTIPLE DISEASES

An inherent problem of polypharmacy is that by definition it introduces complexity into patient care, and this complexity increases the difficulty of empirical studies. The logistics of empirically submitting to trial analysis all the combinations of possible therapies are prohibitive. Thus, although there may be trial data to separately support the prescription of drugs A and B, there will rarely be trial information as to the combination of A and B; there will be uncertainty as to whether A potentiates, antagonizes, or makes B redundant.[63] The confidence in the trial data is thus reduced. The study of multiple treatments is in its infancy. The authors have attempted to apply logic and mathematical analysis to a problem that otherwise has been addressed only qualitatively and heuristically.[64,65]

In the context of independent diseases and treatments (eg, the treatment of bowel cancer with chemotherapy and the anticoagulation of a patient with atrial fibrillation) the authors have shown that the benefits of treatment are always less than those predicted from studies of each condition. This result can be appreciated in simple terms by considering the example discussed previously—some of the benefit of successful bowel cancer chemotherapy will be lost in those patients who suffer a stroke, and alternatively sparing a patient an atrial fibrillation–related stroke loses some of its value if that same patient develops metastatic cancer.

The authors also showed that that an individual treatment may in a trial seem to be cost-effective on account of other therapies that may or may not be cost-effective. A simple example demonstrating this point would be commencement of dialysis in a patient with an implantable defibrillator in situ. Examination of life prolongation of each therapy would show a positive result—each result is, however, dependent on the other, leading to double counting. If dialysis and the defibrillator each prolong life 1 year, it may be that each 1 year is the same year, not a sum equaling 2 years. The cost, on the other hand, is the sum of the costs of the two therapies.

Thus, there are mathematical limitations that apply to trial data in the context of multiple comorbidities. These limitations seem to always inflate the seeming benefit/ risk/cost ratios of individual therapies. It follows that the rationale of following a guideline breaks down in the context of multiple guidelines. The authors have suggested that an intuitive appreciation of these mathematical relationships may underlie the "clinical expertise and judgement" mentioned previously and that further studies might expand this understanding.

WAYS OF DECREASING POLYPHARMACY WITHOUT TENSION WITH GUIDELINES

Not all reductions in polypharmacy come at the cost of sacrificing an intervention supported by trial data and guidelines.[66] Before considering this step there should be a review of the medication list, checking other options. These options include removal of medications that may have been prescribed in error and medications for which the indication may have expired. For example, a patient may be on antiangina medication despite not having had angina for some months—this absence of angina in turn may be due to another problem such as decrease in mobility.

The medication list review should include checking the possibility that some drugs are redundant (eg, two drugs from the same class, or even two identical drugs with different names) or that one drug is being used to treat a side effect of another (eg, frusemide for edema induced by a calcium channel blocker). Drugs that are already

Table 1			
Strategies for resolving the dilemma of polypharmacy versus clinical guidelines			
Elicitation of patient preferences	• Individualize benefit-to-risk ratio in terms of patient values.		
	• Order priorities.		
Use of low-dose therapy	↓ Benefit	}	Improve benefit-to-risk ratio.
	↓↓ Risk		
Formal/heuristic mathematical analysis	• Individualize benefit to risk ratio by mathematical consideration of the effects of age and comorbidities.		
	• Order priorities.		

causing side effects can often be stopped; it is first necessary to actively consider the possibility that any of the patient's difficulties may be drug-related rather than automatically ascribing them to illnesses or the aging process (eg, lethargy due to beta-blockade). N-of-1 trials may help in determining whether or not a particular medication is symptomatically helpful/harmful.[67]

Some problems of polypharmacy may be reduced by the use of combination drugs. In particular, these formulations may assist with expense and adherence. There is a trade-off with flexibility of dosing, and care must be taken to avoid doubling therapy; for example, a patient may be receiving a diuretic incorporated in an antihypertensive and then be prescribed another diuretic. The use of combination drugs does not address the fundamental issue of patients' exposure to multiple therapies and risks.

GUIDELINES VERSUS POLYPHARMACY

Despite all the previously described steps, there will often be residual issues of polypharmacy that necessitate a cognitive analysis and a judgement of risk and benefit. The authors have identified three ways to address this dilemma: the elicitation of patient preferences, the use of low-dose therapy ('mini-polypharmacy'), and formal/heuristic mathematical analysis of the drug and comorbidity list. **Table 1** summarizes these strategies.

Patients' perspectives of their treatments may be quite variable. As discussed previously, the authors' work shows that merely explaining to the patient the absolute risks and benefits of an intervention will lead many patients to dismiss the intervention as not worthwhile. The authors believe that expressing the risk in absolute terms is the preferred option; certainly, expressing benefit in relative terms often gives a more favorable impression, particularly if risks are left in absolute terms. Different impressions may be given by expressing survival versus mortality, and so forth.

Apart from this assessment of risk/benefit, patients in different circumstances may have different priorities. Thus, for one patient a small chance at prolongation of life may be particularly worthwhile, whereas another patient may have greater concern for symptomatic benefit. In these circumstances some medications might be withdrawn on account of the reduced value, from the patient's perspective, of the putative benefits.

Dimmitt and Stampfer[68] have suggested an interesting method of increasing the benefit and safety of polypharmacy. They proposed that small doses be used as possible on the grounds that with increasing doses of medications, the incremental benefit diminishes, whereas the risk of side effects increases. One sees this effect, for example, with statin therapy of dyslipidemia. Each doubling of dose leads to the same relative reduction in cholesterol (a progressively smaller decrement with exponential dose increase), and in outcome trials the benefit of high-dose over low-dose statin is very small. Toxicity of statins increases significantly with the dose. In the context of polypharmacy one therefore might avoid high doses of therapy and thereby "treating to target," aiming more for a measurable effect at minimal toxicity. This strategy is still polypharmacy but in a reduced form—perhaps it might be termed "mini-polypharmacy." The end result is less benefit of therapy but proportionally a greater reduction in risk and cost, leading to an improved benefit/risk/cost ratio.

The mathematical models the authors have explored can also be used to examine the benefits of any polypharmacy combination. The authors are currently evaluating computerized calculations of revised benefits in the context of comorbidity and, it is hoped, in time such analyses will be available for clinicians in practice. In the absence of these calculations, however, it is possible for clinicians to use heuristics ("rules of thumb") as guides.

The first consideration in such an exercise is a semiquantitative estimate as to the risk/benefit of an intervention under normal circumstances. In general terms, the benefits of any treatment are proportional to baseline risk, which in turn is proportional to the extent of any abnormality/risk factor.[3] Thus, treatment of a blood pressure of 220/140 will have more value than treating a blood pressure of 150/90 (at this level any benefit is probably borderline). Treatment of cancer too is likely to have more value than treating mild hypertension. Similarly, secondary prevention usually provides greater benefit than primary prevention; lowering any cholesterol level is more beneficial in the context of previous myocardial infarction.

If we combine these two points, we see that, for example, treating a high cholesterol level in a man with previous myocardial infarction is likely to be beneficial, but treating a lower level in a woman with no history of ischemic heart disease is likely to afford less (if any!) benefit.

Thus, when a list of medications is encountered, one can in semiquantitative terms assign a value to each treatment, for example, strongly indicated down to borderline indication.

The authors have shown that in the context of comorbidity and/or advanced age, the benefits of treatment decline. Therefore, if a given patient is older than or has more severe comorbidity burdens than the index population, we can subtract a proportion from our above assigned values. We can be confident that those treatments that had borderline indications are even less indicated; in other words, benefit is not sufficient to justify ongoing treatment and medications are candidates for withdrawal. Alternatively, one might rank the treatments and withdraw an arbitrary number. Alternatively again, one might choose to continue with polypharmacy, accepting the reduced benefit/risk.

Similar heuristics may be used to analyze the risks and costs of any intervention. In this way one might accept a medication of borderline benefit if it were cheap and well-tolerated, and rather withdraw another medication of perhaps a little greater benefit but associated with significant negative characteristics.

All of the techniques discussed previously may be used in combination. One might combine the assessment of patients' perceptions of benefit/risk and their priorities, with a heuristic model of risk/benefit, and choose to reduce doses rather than withdraw medications altogether when the indication is at best borderline.

The sum total of the previous discussion is a form of decision-analysis. Decision-analysis has often been used to refine the application of treatments to populations of different ages, stage of disease, and so forth. Such decision-analyses generally confirm that benefit is reduced in the context of co morbidity.[69,70] The data and conclusions of trials are thus not the final arbiter as to the place of treatment but are subject to further modeling and modulation. Most decision-analyses are, however, limited in that they consider options for one condition in one direction rather than how the onset of this condition might affect other conditions/treatments.

It is not possible to be dogmatic with regard to most of the treatment of any individual. Most components of polypharmacy are rather prescribed on the basis of probability, and often it is only in retrospect that the possible benefit of a treatment can be partially judged. But even, for example, if a patient has a major stroke that might have been prevented with more vigorous antihypertensive or anticoagulant therapy, one never knows whether that patient might not have suffered an adverse outcome with/because of therapy.

We do know, however, that most of our therapies are associated with only a small chance of benefit and that withdrawal of medications in the context of polypharmacy can lead to improved outcomes.[71] Therefore, addressing polypharmacy, as previously discussed, and potentially in other ways, although theoretically exposing the patient to more risk from disease, is likely to lead to a net benefit and should be a sign of good practice.

The principles enumerated in this article apply also to assessments made away from the bedside for an individual patient. In the context of communities having finite resources, it may be that resources might be diverted from multiple medical interventions, (given that estimates of their value in isolation are greater than the "true" value in the community in the usual context of comorbidity), to higher standard accommodation and supportive care. With more sophisticated analyses it should be possible to quantitate the respective costs and benefits.

Similarly, it follows that much of the literature on quality care may be invalid. This literature predominantly consists of evaluation of the extent to which patients are treated for individual conditions according to guidelines.[2–4] In the absence of consideration of comorbidity, these evaluations overestimate the benefits and underestimate the cost and risk of guideline therapy. It is relatively easy to do the evaluations as they stand as compared with the complex considerations, which are demanded in the context of polypharmacy and comorbidity. Thus, the mechanisms for assessing quality of care need review.

The evaluation of new technology as to whether its introduction can be justified is, again, traditionally made in isolation.[72] A more sophisticated evaluation requires consideration of context according to the same principles as previously discussed.

The ever-increasing number of trials generating data, which is the food for metaanalysis, clinical guidelines, quality assessment, and so forth, has generated the need for a science devoted to the understanding of how these data interact and thus affect patient therapy. This science, not even as yet named, is in its infancy, unlike the patients most in need of it.

REFERENCES

1. DeMets DL, Califf RM. Lessons learned from recent cardiovascular clinical trials: part I. Circulation 2002;106:746–51.
2. Seeman E, Kotowicz MA, Nash PT, et al. Inappropriate prescribing for osteoporosis. Med J Aust 2009;191:355–6.
3. Tonkin AM, Boyden AN, Colagiuri S. Maximising the effectiveness and cost effectiveness of cardiovascular disease prevention in the general population. Med J Aust 2009;191:300–2.

4. Webster JR, Heeley EL, Peiris DP, et al. Gaps in cardiovascular disease risk management in Australian general practice. Med J Aust 2009;191:324–9.
5. Medi C, Hankey GJ, Freedman SB. Atrial fibrillation. Med J Aust 2007;186:197–202.
6. Boyd CM, Darer J, Boult C, et al. Clinical practice guidelines and quality of care for older patients with multiple comorbid diseases. JAMA 2005;294:716–24.
7. Chutka DS, Takahashi PY, Hoel RW. Inappropriate medication use in the elderly. Essent Psychopharmacol 2005;6:331–40.
8. Hilmer NH. The dilemma of polypharmacy. Australian Prescriber 2009;31:2–3.
9. Grimmsmann T, Himmel W. Polypharmacy in primary care practices: an analysis using a large health insurance database. Pharmacoepidemiol Drug Saf 2009;18:1206–13.
10. Dong L, Yan H, Wang D. Polypharmacy and its correlates in village health clinics across 10 provinces of Western China. J Epidemiol Community Health 2010;64:549–53.
11. Garrido-Garrido EM, Garcia-Garrido I, Garcia-Lopez-Duran JC, et al. [Study of polymedicated patients over 65 years-old in an urban primary care centre]. Rev Calid Asist 2011;26:90–6 [in Spanish].
12. Carpenter I, Gambassi G, Topinkova E, et al. Community care in Europe. The Aged in Home Care project (AdHOC). Aging Clin Exp Res 2004;16:259–69.
13. Fialova D, Onder G. Medication errors in elderly people: contributing factors and future perspectives. Br J Clin Pharmacol 2009;67:641–5.
14. Bushardt RL, Massey EB, Simpson TW, et al. Polypharmacy: misleading, but manageable. Clin Interv Aging 2008;3:383–9.
15. Harugeri A, Joseph J, Parthasarathi G, et al. Potentially inappropriate medication use in elderly patients: a study of prevalence and predictors in two teaching hospitals. J Postgrad Med 2010;56:186–91.
16. Bongue B, Naudin F, Laroche ML, et al. Trends of the potentially inappropriate medication consumption over 10 years in older adults in the East of France. Pharmacoepidemiol Drug Saf 2009;18:1125–33.
17. Nobili A, Franchi C, Pasina L, et al. Drug utilization and polypharmacy in an Italian elderly population: the EPIFARM-elderly project. Pharmacoepidemiol Drug Saf 2011;20:488–96.
18. Zink M, Englisch S, Meyer-Lindenberg A. [Polypharmacy in schizophrenia]. Nervenarzt 2010;82:853–8 [in German].
19. Crentsil V, Ricks MO, Xue QL, et al. A pharmacoepidemiologic study of community-dwelling, disabled older women: factors associated with medication use. Am J Geriatr Pharmacother 2010;8:215–24.
20. Dalakishvili S, Bakuradze N, Gugunishvili M, et al. Treatment characteristics in elderly. Georgian Med News 2010:48–51.
21. Aparasu RR, Mort JR, Brandt H. Polypharmacy trends in office visits by the elderly in the United States, 1990 and 2000. Res Social Adm Pharm 2005;1:446–59.
22. Beard K. Drugs in the elderly–more good than harm? Expert Opin Drug Saf 2007;6:229–31.
23. Steinman MA, Landefeld CS, Rosenthal GE, et al. Polypharmacy and prescribing quality in older people. J Am Geriatr Soc 2006;54:1516–23.
24. Avorn J, Gurwitz JH, Rochon PA. Principles of pharmacology. In: Cassel CK, editor. Geriatric medicine: an evidence based approach. 4th edition. New York: Springer; 2003. p. 65–82.
25. William BR, Elizabeth ER, Susan JS, et al. Adverse drug events and medication errors in Australia. Int J Qual Health Care 2003;15:i49–59.
26. Beers MH. Explicit criteria for determining potentially inappropriate medication use by the elderly. An update. Arch Intern Med 1997;157:1531–6.

27. Curtis LH, Ostbye T, Sendersky V, et al. Inappropriate prescribing for elderly Americans in a large outpatient population. Arch Intern Med 2004;164:1621–5.

28. Goulding MR. Inappropriate medication prescribing for elderly ambulatory care patients. Arch Intern Med 2004;164:305–12.

29. Lane CJ, Bronskill SE, Sykora K, et al. Potentially inappropriate prescribing in Ontario community-dwelling older adults and nursing home residents. J Am Geriatr Soc 2004;52:861–6.

30. Fick DM, Mion LC, Beers MH, et al. Health outcomes associated with potentially inappropriate medication use in older adults. Res Nurs Health 2008;31:42–51.

31. Cannon KT, Choi MM, Zuniga MA. Potentially inappropriate medication use in elderly patients receiving home health care: a retrospective data analysis. Am J Geriatr Pharmacother 2006;4:134–43.

32. Fick DM, Cooper JW, Wade WE, et al. Updating the Beers criteria for potentially inappropriate medication use in older adults: results of a US consensus panel of experts. Arch Intern Med 2003;163.

33. Akazawa M, Imai H, Igarashi A, et al. Potentially inappropriate medication use in elderly Japanese patients. Am J Geriatr Pharmacother 2010;8:146–60.

34. Ay P, Akici A, Harmanc H. Drug utilization and potentially inappropriate drug use in elderly residents of a community in Istanbul, Turkey. Int J Clin Pharmacol Ther 2005;43:195–202.

35. Carey IM, De Wilde S, Harris T, et al. What factors predict potentially inappropriate primary care prescribing in older people? Analysis of UK primary care patient record database. Drugs Aging 2008;25:693–706.

36. George J, Phun YT, Bailey MJ, et al. Development and validation of the medication regimen complexity index. Ann Pharmacother 2004;38:1369–76.

37. Melchiors AC, Correr CJ, Fernandez-Llimos F. Translation and validation into Portuguese language of the medication regimen complexity index. Arq Bras Cardiol 2007;89:210–8.

38. Ferrari CM, Castro LH, Settervall CH, et al. Validity and reliability of the Portuguese version of the Epilepsy Medication Treatment Complexity Index for Brazil. Epilepsy Behav 2011;21:467–72.

39. Stange D, Kriston L, Langebrake C, et al. Development and psychometric evaluation of the German version of the Medication Regimen Complexity Index (MRCI-D). J Eval Clin Pract 2011. [Epub ahead of print].

40. Acurcio Fde A, Silva AL, Ribeiro AQ, et al. [Complexity of therapeutic regimens prescribed for elderly retirees, Belo Horizonte/MG, Brazil]. Rev Assoc Med Bras 2009;55:468–74 [in Portuguese].

41. Briesacher BA, Gurwitz JH, Soumerai SB. Patients at-risk for cost-related medication nonadherence: a review of the literature. J Gen Intern Med 2007;22:864–71.

42. Cardenas-Valladolid J, Martin-Madrazo C, Salinero-Fort MA, et al. Prevalence of adherence to treatment in homebound elderly people in primary health care: a descriptive, cross-sectional, multicentre study. Drugs Aging 2010;27:641–51.

43. Browne T, Merighi JR. Barriers to adult hemodialysis patients' self-management of oral medications. Am J Kidney Dis 2010;56:547–57.

44. Boult C, Altmann M, Gilbertson D, et al. Decreasing disability in the 21st century: the future effects of controlling six fatal and nonfatal conditions. Am J Public Health 1996;86:1388–93.

45. Nancy E. Schoenberg HK, Edwards W, et al. Burden of common multiple-morbidity constellations on out-of-pocket medical expenditures among older adults. Gereotologist 2007;47:423–47.

46. Public health. European Union, 1995–2011. Available at: http://ec.europa.eu/health/major_chronic_diseases/diseases/index_en.htm. Accessed July 22, 2011.

47. Health of older people in Australia: A snapshot, 2004–05 Australian Bureau of Statistics, 2006. Available at: http://www.abs.gov.au/ausstats/abs.nsf/mf/4833.0.55.001/. Accessed November 10, 2011.

48. Santos-Eggimann B. [Population health profile at the age of 65–70]. Rev Med Suisse 2007;3:2546–8, 2550–1 [in French].

49. Bowling A, Mariotto A, Evans O. Are older people willing to give up their place in the queue for cardiac surgery to a younger person? Age Ageing 2002;31:187–92.

50. Kass-Bartelmes BL. Preventing disability in the elderly with chronic disease. Agency for Healthcare Research and Quality. Research in Action 2002;3:1–8. Available at: http://www.ahrq.gov/research/elderdis.pdf. Accessed January 11, 2012.

51. Coory MD. Ageing and healthcare costs in Australia: a case of policy-based evidence? Med J Aust 2004;180:581–3.

52. Fries JF. Aging, natural death, and the compression of morbidity. 1980. Bull World Health Organ 2002;80:245–50.

53. Thomas EJ, Brennan TA. Incidence and types of preventable adverse events in elderly patients: population based review of medical records. BMJ 2000;380:741–4.

54. Jahnigen D, Hannon C, Laxson L, et al. Iatrogenic disease in hospitalized elderly veterans. J Am Geriatr Soc 1982;30:387–90.

55. Riedinger JL, Robbins LJ. Prevention of iatrogenic illness: adverse drug reactions and nosocomial infections in hospitalized older adults. Clin Geriatr Med 1998;14:681–98.

56. Rossi MI, Young A, Maher R, et al. Polypharmacy and health beliefs in older outpatients. Am J Geriatr Pharmacother 2007;5:317–23.

57. Rolita L, Freedman M. Over-the-counter medication use in older adults. J Gerontol Nurs 2008;34:8–17.

58. Walley T. Lifestyle medicines and the elderly. Drugs Aging 2002;19:163–8.

59. Scott IA, Guyatt GH. Cautionary tales in the interpretation of clinical studies involving older persons. Arch Intern Med 2010;170:587–95.

60. Sackett DL, Rosenberg WM, Gray JA, et al. Evidence based medicine: what it is and what it isn't. BMJ 1996;312:71–7.

61. Fitzgerald SP, Phillipov G. Patient attitudes to commonly promoted medical interventions. Med J Aust 2000;172:9–12.

62. Preskorn SH, Lacey RL. Polypharmacy: when is it rational? J Psychiatr Pract 2007; 13:97–105.

63. Califf RM, DeMets DL. Principles from clinical trials relevant to clinical practice. Circulation 2002;106:1172–5.

64. Fitzgerald SP. The overall benefits risks and costs of multiple interventions may be less favourable than the sum of the benefits risks and costs of those individual interventions. Med Hypotheses 2007;69:970–3.

65. Fitzgerald SP, Bean NG. An analysis of the interactions between individual comorbidities and their treatments–implications for guidelines and polypharmacy. J Am Med Dir Assoc 2010;11:475–84.

66. Morley JE, Tumosa N. Conundrums of polypharmacy. Aging Successfully. A newsletter of the Division of Geriatric Medicine, Department of Internal Medicine, Saint Louis University School of Medicine; Geriatric Research, Education and Clinical Center, St Louis Veterans Administration Medical Center; and the Gateway Geriatric Education Center of Missouri and Illinois. Summer 2003.

67. Gabler NB, Duan N, Vohra S, et al. N-of-1 trials in the medical literature: a systematic review. Med Care 2011;49:761–8.

68. Dimmitt SB, Stampfer HG. Low drug doses may improve outcomes in chronic diseases. Med J Aust 2009;191:511–3.

69. Jassal SV, Krahn MD, Naglie G, et al. Kidney transplantation in the elderly: a decision analysis. J Am Soc Nephrol 2003;14:187–96.

70. Nagaki T, Sato K, Yoshida T, et al. Benefit of carotid endarterectomy for symptomatic and asymptomatic severe carotid artery stenosis: a Markov model based on data from randomized controlled trials. J Neurosurg 2009;111:970–7.

71. Polypharmacy interventions result in sustained decreases. Manag Care 2005;14:56.

72. Sanders GD, Hlatky MA, Owens DK. Cost-effectiveness of implantable cardioverter-defibrillators. N Engl J Med 2005;353:1471–80.

Factors Associated With Polypharmacy in Nursing Home Residents

Bruce K. Tamura, MD*, Christina L. Bell, MD, MS,
Michiko Inaba, MD, PhD, Kamal H. Masaki, MD

KEYWORDS

- Long-term care • Nursing home • Polypharmacy
- Comorbidities • Associated factors

Which long-term care patients are at risk for polypharmacy? Are there certain populations that we should target to reduce polypharmacy? The nursing home population has one of the highest rates of polypharmacy, with prevalence rates ranging from 14% to 24% depending on the definition of polypharmacy used ($\geq$10 medications or $\geq$9 medications, respectively).[1,2] Nursing home patients use the highest number of medications compared with the noninstitutionalized elderly.[3] There are few systematic reviews of factors associated with polypharmacy in long-term care. This summary of the literature on factors associated with polypharmacy in nursing homes is aimed toward clinicians practicing in long-term care.

METHODS

We performed a MEDLINE search using the words polypharmacy, medication, nursing home, and long-term care. We reviewed only English-language articles starting from 1990. We included only original articles specific to nursing homes and excluded nursing home articles that included home-bound patients, outpatients, assisted living, or hospital settings.

There are many definitions of polypharmacy in the literature, including number of medications or use of inappropriate medications. In this review, we included data on polypharmacy defined by number of medications used and excluded information on inappropriate medication use, which was considered a separate subject area, and not covered in this review. We extracted the data from articles systematically using standardized tables. Data were sorted by size of study and types of factors associated with polypharmacy.

The John A. Hartford Center of Excellence in Geriatrics, Department of Geriatric Medicine, John A. Burns School of Medicine, University of Hawaii, 347 North Kuakini Street, HPM-9 Honolulu, HI 96817, USA
* Corresponding author.
E-mail address: bktamura@hotmail.com

Clin Geriatr Med 28 (2012) 199–216
doi:10.1016/j.cger.2012.01.004
0749-0690/12/$ – see front matter © 2012 Elsevier Inc. All rights reserved.

RESULTS
Demographic Factors

Age

There is controversy in the literature about the association between age and polypharmacy. Some studies have found no significant association, whereas others have found that older age is associated with lower numbers of medications **(Table 1)**.

The largest negative study was by Gupta and colleagues,[4] who studied 19,932 patients in Louisiana intermediate care facilities in 1994. Using state Medicaid claim history and drug files, they found no significant difference between age groups (65–70, 71–75, 76–80, 81–85, 86–90, 91–95, and >96 years) and number of drugs prescribed. Three other studies found no significant association between age and number of medications prescribed. Bergman and associates[5] performed a cross-sectional study of 7904 patients in Sweden in 2003, using data on all prescribed drugs from the Swedish national register for multidose users. There was no difference in the average number of drugs prescribed per person among those who were 65 to 79 years of age and those who were 80 years or older (11.9 in both). Chiang and co-workers[6] performed a chart review of 414 patients in nursing homes in 3 states. Age was not a predictor of number of routine medications in their bivariate analysis. Chen and colleagues[7] performed a retrospective chart review of 31 patients in 1 nursing home, and found no association between age and total number of medications.

Some studies showed a significant decrease in number of medications with increased age. The largest study used data from a National Nursing Home Survey of 13,403 United States nursing home patients by Dwyer and co-workers[8] in 2004. Information was collected during a face-to-face interview with a designated nursing home respondent who obtained the data from patient medication administration records. Patients 85 years of age or older had the lowest percentage (34.8%) of polypharmacy defined as concurrent use of 9 or more medications. Olsson and associates[9] used a computerized national pharmacy drug register in Sweden to study 2938 nursing home patients in 2002. Patients 80 years and older had a significantly lower number of drugs prescribed compared with those who were 65 to 79 years of age. Elseviers and colleagues[10] performed a retrospective chart review of 2510 patients randomly selected from a random sample of 76 Belgian nursing homes in 2002. Nurse researchers obtained a copy of the medication chart and used a special data entry program to transfer the data into a computerized database. There was a borderline significant linear relationship between age and number of chronic medications prescribed. Beers and colleagues[11] conducted a prospective, 1-month study of 1106 patients in 12 skilled nursing facilities in California between 1990 and 1991, and found that patients 85 years of age and older were ordered fewer medications than those 65 to 84 years (6.9 vs 7.5 drugs). Regression analysis showed that for each decade of age over 65 years, patients were ordered approximately 0.3 fewer medications. Balogun and co-workers[12] performed a cross-sectional study on 175 patients in 2 Virginia nursing homes in 2002, and found that a higher percentage of patients younger than 85 years (43.4%) compared with those 85 years or older (30.4%) were taking 12 or more medications. Wayne and co-workers[13] conducted a chart review of 81 new skilled nursing facility/intermediate care facility patients from July 1988 through July 1989 in New Mexico, and found that age in years was inversely associated with number of scheduled medications and total medications.

Table 1
Demographic factors associated with polypharmacy in nursing home patients

Author and Year	Study Population, Setting, Year and Data Source	Results
Age		
Gupta[4] 1996	n = 19,932 patients in Louisiana NH 1994, Medicaid claim and drug files	Age not significantly associated with number of meds: $P = .4216$
Dwyer[8] 2010	n = 13,403 US NH residents 2004, NNHS	Increased age associated with lower likelihood of polypharmacy: Age ≥ 85; OR, 0.67 (95% CI, 0.57–0.79); age 75–84; OR, 0.98 (95% CI, 0.8–1.16); age 65–74; OR, 1.06 (95% CI, 0.88–1.29); age <65, reference
Bergman[5] 2007	n = 7904 patients in Sweden NH 2003, cross-sectional, drug register	Age not significantly associated with number of meds: Age 65–79 years, mean, 11.9 meds per patient; age ≥80, mean 11.9 meds per patient; $P = .96$
Olsson[9] 2010	n = 3705 patients in 2 Swedish counties NH 2002, drug register	Increased age associated with lower number of meds: Age 65–79, mean 11.2 meds per patient; age ≥80, mean 10.4 meds per patient; $P<.001$
Elseviers[10] 2010	n = 2510 patients randomly selected sample in 76 Belgian NH 2005, retrospective chart review	Increased age borderline associated with lower number of meds; $P = .062$
Beers[11] 1992	n = 1106 patients in 12 SNF in California, 1990–1991, prospective data collection over 1-month period	Increased age associated with lower number of meds: Age 65–84, mean 7.5meds per patient vs age ≥85, mean 6.9 meds per patient; $P<.01$
Chiang[6] 2000	n = 414 patients at 20 NH in 3 states, chart review	Age not significantly associated with number of meds; $P = $ NS
Balogun[12] 2005	n = 175 patients in 2 Virginia NH 2002, cross-sectional admission dataset	Age <85 years, 43.4% took ≥12 medications vs age ≥85, 30.4% took ≥12 medications; $P = .042$
Wayne[13] 1992	n = 81 all new SNF/ICF NH patients in New Mexico 1988–1989, chart review	Increased age associated with lower number of meds: Spearman coefficient −0.37, $P = .0007$; $P = .003$ on linear regression model
Chen[7] 2010	n = 31 patients in 1 NH, retrospective chart review	Age not significantly associated with number of meds; $P = .51$

(continued on next page)

Table 1
(continued)

Author and Year	Study Population, Setting, Year and Data Source	Results
Gender		
Gupta[4] 1996	n = 19,932 patients in Louisiana NH 1994, Medicaid claim and drug files	Gender not significantly associated with number of meds; $P = .9503$
Dwyer[8] 2010	n = 13,403 US NH residents 2004, NNHS	Female gender significantly associated with polypharmacy (≥ 9 meds): Adjusted OR, 1.10 (95% CI, 1.00–1.20)
Bergman[5] 2007	n = 7904 patients in Sweden NH 2003, cross-sectional, drug register	Female gender had borderline association with more meds: Males, 11.8 meds per patient vs females, 12.0 meds per patient; $P = .07$
Elseviers[10] 2010	n = 2510 patients randomly selected sample in 76 Belgian NH 2005, retrospective chart review	Gender not significantly associated with number of meds
Beers[11] 1992	n = 1106 patients in 12 SNF in California, 1990–1991, prospective data collection over a 1-month period	Female gender associated with more meds: Females, 7.3 meds per patient vs males, 6.6 meds per patient; $P<.002$
Balogun[12] 2005	n = 175 patients in 2 Virginia NH 2002, cross-sectional admission dataset	Gender not significantly associated with polypharmacy (≥ 12 meds): Females, 40.8% on ≥ 12 meds vs males, 38.9% on ≥ 12 meds; $P = .463$
Wayne[13] 1992	n = 81 all new SNF/ICF NH patients in New Mexico 1988–1989, chart review	Males prescribed more scheduled meds vs females; males, 4.4 mean scheduled meds per patient vs females, 3.0 mean scheduled meds per patient; $P<.05$; no significant difference in total number of medications by gender
Chen[7] 2010	n = 31 patients in 1 NH, retrospective chart review	Gender not significantly associated with total number of medications; $P = .79$
Race and other factors		
Gupta[4] 1996	n = 19,932 patients in Louisiana NH 1994, Medicaid claim and drug files	Race significantly associated with total number of medications: White vs African American, $P = .0001$; other ethnicity vs African American, $P = .0010$

Dwyer[8] 2010	n = 13,403 US NH residents 2004, NNHS	Race significantly associated with polypharmacy (≥9 meds): Black/other vs white, adjusted OR, 0.80 (95% CI, 0.69–0.93)
Hanlon[14] 2009	n = 3480 patients in veteran NH 2004–2005, VA database	Race not significantly associated with polypharmacy (≥9 meds), $P = .62$
Elseviers[10] 2010	n = 2510 patients randomly selected sample in 76 Belgian NH 2005, retrospective chart review	Socioeconomic status not significantly associated with amount of chronic medications used

Abbreviations: CI, confidence interval; NH, nursing home; NNHS, National Nursing Home Survey; OR, odds ratio.

Table 2
Function and disease factors associated with polypharmacy in nursing home patients

Author and Year	Study Population, Setting, Year and Data Source	Results
Landi[19] 1998	n = 260,628 NH patients in 5 states 1992–1995, Medicaid/Medicare Minimum Data Set data cross-sectional	Cognitive impairment significantly associated with lower average number of meds: Severe cognitive impairment, 5.9 meds per patient; moderate cognitive impairment, 6.2 meds per patient; normal, 7.3 meds per patient
Dwyer[8] 2010	n = 13,403 US NH residents 2004, NNHS	Number of comorbidities significantly associated with polypharmacy (≥9 meds): 4–6 comorbidities, aOR, 1.57 (95% CI, 1.36–1.81); 7–9 comorbidities, aOR, 2.70 (95% CI, 2.32–3.15); ≥10 comorbidities, aOR, 5.18 (95% CI, 4.36–6.15); reference, ≤3 comorbidities
Elseviers[10] 2010	n = 2510 patients randomly selected sample in 76 Belgian NH 2005, retrospective chart review	Number of diagnoses associated with number of chronic medications: r = 0.496, $P<.001$; number of geriatric syndromes [a] associated with number of chronic medications: rs = 0.308, $P<0.001$; depression associated with number of chronic medications, depression (mean 8.6 meds per patient) vs no depression (mean 6.3 meds per patient; $P<.001$); dementia inversely associated with number of chronic medications, dementia (mean 4.9 meds per patient) vs no dementia (mean 7.7 meds per patient; $P<.001$)
Hosia-Randell[21] 2008	n = 1987 patients in Finland NH 2003, chart review	Dementia associated with less polypharmacy (>9 meds), $P<.001$; stroke associated with more polypharmacy, $P<.001$; depression associated with more polypharmacy, P = .001; poor nutrition associated with less polypharmacy, $P<.01$; psychotropic medication associated with more polypharmacy, $P<.001$
Nygaard[22] 2003	n = 1042 patients in 15 Norwegian NHs 1996–1997, Pharmacy data	Cognitive impairment inversely associated with number of meds: Cognitively impaired (mean 4.8 meds per patient) vs normal (mean 6.2 meds per patient; $P<.001$)

Study	Sample	Findings
Chiang[6] 2000	n = 414 patients at 20 NH in 3 states, chart review	Number of diagnoses associated with total number of meds, $P<.05$; cognitive impairment inversely associated with total number of meds, $P<.001$; CHF, hypertension, anxiety, depression and diabetes each associated with total number of meds—CHF ($P<.001$), hypertension ($P<.05$), anxiety ($P<.001$), depression ($P<.05$), diabetes ($P<.05$); cancer not significantly associated with total number of meds
Balogun[12] 2005	n = 175 patients in 2 Virginia NH 2002, cross-sectional admission dataset	Dementia borderline inversely associated with polypharmacy: Dementia, 27.8% on ≥12 meds; 72.2% on <12 meds ($P = .067$); psychotropic medication not associated with polypharmacy, taking psychotropic meds: 43.6% on ≥12 meds, 56.4% on <12 meds ($P = .105$)
Wayne[13] 1992	n = 81 all new SNF/ICF NH patients in New Mexico 1988–1989, chart review	Number of diagnoses significantly associated with number of scheduled meds ($r = 0.25$; $P = .02$) and borderline significant association with number of total meds ($r = 0.20$; $P = .07$); mental status score not associated with number of scheduled meds ($r = 0.18$; $P = .20$) or number of total meds ($r = 0.22$; $P = .12$); ADLs not associated with number of scheduled meds ($r = 0.10$; $P = .38$) or number of total meds ($r = 0.07$; $P = .51$)
Chen[7] 2010	n = 31 patients in 1 NH, retrospective chart review	Heart disease associated with total number of meds ($P = .04$); gastrointestinal disease borderline associated with total number of meds ($P = .05$); other diseases (lung disease, hypertension, diabetes, stroke, cancer, psychiatric disease) not associated with total number of meds ($P>.05$)

Abbreviations: ADL, activities of daily living; aOR, adjusted odds ratio; CHF, congestive heart failure; CI, confidence interval; NNHS, National Nursing Home Survey.
[a] Geriatric Syndromes: in original paper these were described as care problems and included risk of falling, insomnia, constipation, incontinence and chronic pain.

Gender

Studies have found mixed results about the association of gender with polypharmacy. Some studies have shown no significant association. Gupta and colleagues[4] found no difference in polypharmacy by gender, using Medicaid data from 19,932 patients in Louisiana intermediate care facilities. Elseviers and associates[10] showed no gender differences in the number of chronic medications prescribed in nursing homes in Belgium. Balogun and co-workers[12] found that a higher percentage of female patients (40.8%) compared with male patients (38.9%) were taking 12 or more medications, but this difference was not significant. Chen and colleagues[7] found no association between gender and total number of medications.

A few studies found a significant association between gender and polypharmacy. Dwyer and associates[8] used the 2004 National Nursing Home Survey and showed that female patients had slightly higher odds of receiving polypharmacy ($\geq$9 medications; odds ratio [OR], 1.10; 95% confidence interval [CI], 1.00–1.20). Bergman and colleagues[5] showed borderline differences, with females prescribed a greater average number of drugs per person. Beers and associates[11] showed that women were prescribed more medications (7.3 drugs compared with 6.6 in men) in a 1-month, prospective study in California. Only 1 small study in 81 new nursing home admissions found that males were prescribed more scheduled medications than females (4.4 vs 3.0 respectively).[13]

Race/other factors

We found 3 studies that looked at the association between race and polypharmacy, with mixed results. Gupta and co-workers[4] used Medicaid data and delineated race into White (n = 14,081), African-American (n = 4627), or other (n = 1224), and found that the number of drugs prescribed was positively correlated with White or other race, compared with African-American race. Using data from the 2004 National Nursing Home Survey, Dwyer and associates[8] found that Black/other race patients had lower odds of receiving polypharmacy (OR, 0.80; 95% CI, 0.69–0.93) compared with Whites. Hanlon and colleagues[14] studied a Veterans Affairs database of 3480 patients across the United States from 2004 to 2005, and found that Blacks were as likely as Whites to take 9 or more medications (74.35% vs 71.18%, respectively). Only 1 study in 76 Belgian nursing homes conducted by Elseviers and co-workers[10] looked at socioeconomic status with relation to polypharmacy, and found that administrative status of underprivileged patients did not influence the amount of chronic medications used.

Functional Status and Chronic Disease Factors

Cognitive function

Dementia is a prevalent, devastating, and costly disease affecting many elderly persons in the United States. It is estimated that nearly 75% of all persons with dementia will eventually be admitted to a nursing home.[15] The prevalence of dementia in nursing homes is estimated to be 48.2% to 54.5% in the United States,[16,17] and about 11% of residents diagnosed with dementia have severe cognitive impairment (Table 2).[18]

The majority of studies of cognitive function and polypharmacy found that cognitive impairment or dementia was associated with use of lower number of medications. Landi and colleagues[19] performed a cross-sectional study of 260,628 patients using the Medicaid/Medicare Minimum Data Set in5 states between 1992 and 1995. The average number of medications was significantly lower among patients with moderate and severe cognitive impairment (6.2 $\pm$ 4.3 and 5.9 $\pm$ 4.6, respectively) compared with cognitively normal patients (7.3 ± 4.4). Elseviers and associates[10] studied nursing home patients in Belgium, using the Katz scale, which evaluates dementia using a 5-stage grading system to judge disorientation in time and place, ranging from "cognitively fit" to "full dependence and dementia."[20] They found the number of chronic medications steadily decreased with increasing severity of dementia, ranging from a mean of 7.7 ± 3.6 in mentally healthy patients to 4.9 ± 2.6 in patients with complete disorientation to time and place. Hosia-Randell and colleagues[21] did a chart review of 1987 patients in Finland in 2003, and found that patients taking 9 or more drugs were significantly less likely than other patients to have been diagnosed with dementia (95% CI, 0.11–0.19). Nygaard and colleagues[22] used 1996 through 1997 pharmacy data on 1042 patients in 15 Norwegian nursing homes, and found that mentally intact patients used significantly more drugs than mentally impaired patients (6.2 ± 2.6 vs 4.8 ± 2.4, respectively). Chiang and associates[6] conducted a chart review study of 414 patients in 20 nursing homes in 3 states and found that cognitive impairment was associated significantly with lower numbers of routine medications. Balogun and co-workers[12] studied nursing home patients in Virginia, and found that patients taking fewer than 12 medications were more likely to have a diagnosis of dementia compared with those taking 12 or more medications (72.2% vs 27.8%). Wayne and colleagues[13] reviewed patient chart mental status scores as defined by the Mini-Mental Status Exam for new nursing home admissions in New Mexico.[23] No association was found between scheduled medications or total medications and mental status score.

Dementia and use of inappropriate medications

Pharmacologic treatment in dementia should be guided by the goals of care. Some medications may have limited benefit among those whose primary goal of care is palliation. Holmes and associates[24] analyzed data from 34 patients with advanced dementia enrolled in the Palliative Excellence in Alzheimer Care Efforts Program. Patients were taking an average of 6.5 medications at enrollment, and 6 patients were taking 10 or more medications daily. Of the 221 medications prescribed at enrollment, 5% were considered to be never appropriate, and 10 of 34 patients (29%) had been taking a medication considered to be never appropriate.

Antipsychotic drugs are widely used to treat psychosis, aggression, and agitation in patients with dementia, but their benefits are uncertain and concerns about safety have been raised. One study using the Medicare Current Beneficiary Survey data for 2000 and 2001 found that the most common indicator for antipsychotic use by Medicare beneficiaries in nursing homes was dementia with aggression.[25] In many nursing homes in Europe and North America, between 25% and 63% of residents with dementia are prescribed antipsychotics, commonly for longer than a year.[26,27]

The evidence for long-term treatment with antipsychotic medications is somewhat lacking. The few studies of antipsychotic drug treatment lasting for 6 months or longer suggest no or only modest benefit from longer duration of therapy. A trial conducted by Ballard and colleagues[26] found that for most patients with Alzheimer disease, withdrawal of antipsychotics had no overall detrimental effect on functional and cognitive status; in fact, by some measures function and cognition improved. After adjusting for the presence of hallucinations or behavioral problems (eg, physical agitation and wandering), the likelihood of being prescribed antipsychotic medications was found to be significantly greater among residents dying with advanced dementia than among those with terminal cancer. It is reported that approximately one quarter (24.9%) of patients with advanced dementia in nursing homes received antipsychotic medications at the end of life.[28] A prospective cohort study of medication usage in nursing home residents with advanced dementia by Blass and co-workers[29] found that, among patients who died during the study, medication use for psychosis fell from 27% at baseline (during the 6 months before study enrollment) to 11% at the final medical record review before death. Randomized, double-blind, placebo-controlled trials in institutionalized patients with severe dementia have not demonstrated worsening behavior after withdrawal of antipsychotics.[26,27,30-32] It has been argued that there is no obvious need for long-term treatment, and that attempts to taper and discontinue antipsychotic agents should be undertaken at regular intervals and in a standardized fashion, with frequent reevaluation of benefits and risks. Thus, antipsychotic medication withdrawal seems to be a rational management option once a patient has stabilized, although data on the clinical effect of antipsychotic withdrawal are somewhat limited and withdrawal symptoms/syndrome, although rare, can be severe.

Gruber-Baldini and colleagues[33] reported on the use of acetylcholinesterase inhibitors by Medicare beneficiaries in long-term care facilities. Among patients prescribed acetylcholinesterase inhibitors, 11.0% had mild dementia, 36.2 % had moderate dementia, and 52.8% had severe dementia. Tjia and co-workers[17] reported that 15.8% of residents with advanced dementia were prescribed acetylcholinesterase inhibitors and 9.9% were prescribed memantine. Reduction of antidementia medications was observed in residents with advanced dementia in nursing homes (14.9%–7.9%), but the reduction happened very close to death. One population-based study found that, on average, acetylcholinesterase inhibitors were used for more than 2 years.[34] More than half the patients died during the observation period, and 30% of patients in long-term care died while receiving acetylcholinesterase inhibitors despite the questionable efficacy of these drugs in this population.

A recent consensus panel listed acetylcholinesterase inhibitors as one of the "never appropriate medications" for individuals with advanced dementia when comfort is the goal of care.[24] Weschules and associates[35] performed a cross-sectional study of 10,065 patients with end-stage dementia admitted to 1 of 441 US hospices in 2004. They reported that 21% of patients were prescribed acetylcholinesterase inhibitors and/or memantine therapy at the time of hospice enrollment. Parsons and colleagues[36] recently reported on 3506 patients with dementia newly admitted to nursing homes in 2006. They found use of acetylcholinesterase inhibitors and memantine on admission was significantly higher in residents with mild to moderately severe dementia, compared with those with advanced dementia (41.2% vs 33.3%). After 3 months of follow-up, use of both classes of drugs decreased significantly (31.1% for mild to moderately severe dementia patients vs 25.6% for advanced dementia patients). Although the study showed a significant decrease in acetylcholinesterase inhibitors and memantine use 3 months after nursing home admission, a large percentage of patients with advanced dementia remained on these medications.

Depression

Studies have found that depression is associated with polypharmacy. Elseviers and co-workers[10] found that the clinical diagnosis of depression in nursing homes in Belgium was associated with a significant increase in the consumption of chronic medications from a mean of 6.3 $\pm$ 3.2 to a mean of 8.6 $\pm$ 3.3. Hosia-Randell and associates[21] used the Resident Assessment Instrument Depression Score with a cut point of 3 or higher (range, 0–14),[37] and found that patients taking 9 or more drugs daily were significantly more likely to have a current depression diagnosis. Chiang and associates[6] found that a diagnosis of depression on chart review was associated with higher numbers of routine and total medications.

Other chronic diseases

Studies of the association of polypharmacy with other chronic diseases have had mixed results. Hosia-Randell and colleagues[21] found that patients in nursing homes in Finland who were taking 9 or more medications daily were more likely to have a past history of stroke. Using the Mini-Nutritional Assessment Score,[38] patients taking 9 or more medications were less likely to have a poor nutritional status, defined as a score below 17. Chiang and associates[6] found that diagnoses of congestive heart failure, hypertension, anxiety, and diabetes mellitus were independently associated with higher numbers of total medications. A cancer diagnosis was not associated with the number of medications. Chen and colleagues[7] found that patients with heart disease were prescribed significantly more medications, but there were no associations between total medication use and lung disease, hypertension, diabetes mellitus, cerebrovascular accident, cancer, psychiatric disease, and gastrointestinal disease.

Several studies have demonstrated a significant association between number of comorbidities and increased number of medications used. Using data from the 2004 National Nursing Home Survey, Dwyer and co-workers[8] found that the percentage of patients who received polypharmacy ($\geq$9 medications) increased with the number of comorbidities, from 24.8% for patients with 3 or fewer comorbidities to 61.9% for patients with 10 or more comorbidities. Elseviers and colleagues[10] reported that the number of chronic medications per patient was strongly associated with the number of clinical problems listed in charts of Belgian nursing home patients. The same Belgian study also found a significant relationship between polypharmacy and increasing care problems (eg, risk for falling, insomnia, constipation, incontinence, chronic pain). Chiang and associates[6] extracted data on diagnoses from the Minimum Data Set and found that the total number of diagnoses was significantly associated with higher numbers of routine medications and total medications. Wayne and co-workers[13] found a significant association between number of diagnoses and number of scheduled medications, but not total medications.

Use of psychotropic medications

Hosia-Randell and colleagues[21] found that patients taking 9 or more medications daily were more likely to be taking psychotropic medications. However, Balogun and associates[12] found no significant difference in psychotropic medication use between patients taking fewer than 12 medications versus patients taking 12 or more medications.

Functional status

There have been few studies of activities of daily living (ADLs) and polypharmacy, with mixed results. Dwyer and associatres[8] used number of ADLs (bathing, dressing, walking, eating, toileting) requiring assistance by nursing home staff ($\leq$4 or all 5) as an independent variable. Patients who received assistance from the nursing home staff with all 5 ADLs had a lower prevalence of polypharmacy ($\geq$9 medications) compared with those who received assistance with 4 or more ADLs (34.9% vs 44.9%). Wayne and colleagues[13] reviewed charts for patients' ADL index,[20] and found no association between ADL score and scheduled medications or total medications.

Systems of Care and Healthcare Financing Factors

Prescribers

Studies have demonstrated that having a greater number of prescribers is associated with increased number of medications used **(Table 3)**. Gupta and collagues[4] found the number of drugs positively correlated with larger numbers of prescribing physicians.

Table 3
Systems of care and financing factors associated with polypharmacy in Nursing Home (NH) patients

Author and Year	Study Population, Setting, Year and Data Source	Results
Gupta[4] 1996	n = 19,932 patients in Louisiana NH 1994, Medicaid claim and drug files	Number of physicians associated with number of meds ($P<.0001$); number of pharmacies associated with number of meds ($P = .0001$)
Dwyer[8] 2010	n = 13,403 US NH residents 2004, NNHS	For profit NH status inversely associated with polypharmacy (≥ 9 meds); aOR, 0.84 (95% CI, 0.75–0.95); reference, not-for-profit NH; number of NH beds inversely associated with polypharmacy (≥ 9 meds): 100–199 beds, aOR, 0.89 (95% CI, 0.81–0.),9; ≥ 200 beds, aOR, 0.74 (95% CI, 0.60–0.91); reference, 3–99 beds; primary payment source associated with polypharmacy (≥ 9 meds), out-of-pocket/private aOR, 0.66 (95% CI, 0.58–0.75); Medicare, unknown, and other insurance, not significant; reference, Medicaid Length of stay associated with polypharmacy (≥ 9 meds): 3 to <6 months aOR, 1.25, 95% CI, 1.04–1.50; 6 months to <5 years not significant; ≥ 5 years aOR, 0.68 (95% CI, 0.56–0.82); reference, <3 months
Bergman[5] 2007	n = 7904 patients in Sweden NH 2003, cross-sectional, drug register	Number of physicians significantly associated with number of meds, OR, 1.40 (95% CI, 1.36–1.45)
Olsson[9] 2010	n = 3705 patients in 2 Swedish counties NH 2002, drug register	Number of prescribers associated with number of meds, OR, 1.22 (95% CI, 1.15–1.29)
Elseviers[10] 2010	n = 2510 patients randomly selected sample in 76 Belgian NH 2005, retrospective chart review	Large public NH inversely associated with number of meds per patient; NH served by a hospital pharmacy associated with lower number of meds per patient ($P = .022$)
Chiang[6] 2000	n = 414 patients at 20 NH in 3 states, chart review	Larger NH inversely associated with total number of meds per patient ($P<.05$)
Arinzon[39] 2006	n = 324 patients in Israel NH 2001–2002, prospective data	No significant difference in number of meds per patient comparing newly admitted patients to those institutionalized for ≥ 3 months (P = NS)

Koopmans[40] 2003	n = 254 patients in 6 Dutch NH 1999–2000, drug database	Patients admitted from home taking lower number of meds compared with those admitted from hospital or residential home: Home, mean of 4.1 meds per patient; hospital, mean of 6.3 meds per patient; residential home, mean of 6.1 meds per patient ($P<.01$)
Balogun[12] 2005	n = 175 patients in 2 Virginia NH 2002, cross-sectional admission dataset	No significant differences in patients taking ≥12 meds when comparing those admitted from home vs those admitted from hospital, rehab, assisted living, or another NH ($P = .242$)
Wayne[13] 1992	n = 81 all new SNF/ICF NH patients in New Mexico 1988–1989, chart review	ICF vs SNF level of NH care not associated with mean number of total meds: Length of stay significantly associated with mean number of total meds, after 3 months mean of 6.2 total meds per patient vs on entry to NH mean of 4.7 total meds per patient ($P<.001$)
Chen[7] 2010	n = 31 patients in 1 NH, retrospective chart review	Length of stay not associated with total number of meds ($P = .86$)

Abbreviations: aOR, adjusted odds ratio; ICF, intermediate care facility; NNHS, National Nursing Home Survey; SNF, skilled nursing facility.

Bergman and co-wrokers[5] showed the average number of physicians prescribing drugs per resident was 3.9 (± 2.1; range, 1–16) and that number of prescribers was positively associated with number of prescribed drugs (OR, 1.40; 95% CI, 1.36–1.45). Olson and colleagues[9] reported the mean number of prescribers was 3.2 (range, 1–14), and found that higher number of prescribers per resident was associated with a higher number of drugs prescribed (OR, 1.22; 95% CI, 1.15–1.29).

Pharmacies
Studies have also demonstrated that the more pharmacies that are used by nursing homes, the greater the number of medications used. Gupta and associates[4] found the number of drugs prescribed was significantly correlated with the use of a larger number of pharmacies. Elseviers and co-workers[10] found that nursing homes served by a hospital pharmacy had lower consumption of chronic medications.

Size of nursing home
Studies have found that size of nursing home is significantly associated with number of medications, with patients in larger nursing homes taking lower number of medications. Dwyer and associates[8] categorized the size of the nursing home to small (3–99 beds), medium (100–199 beds), and large (≥200 beds). Multivariate results showed that the odds of polypharmacy decreased with increasing bed size, from small facilities (OR, 1.00, reference), to medium facilities (OR, 0.89; 95% CI, 0.81–0.99), to large facilities (OR, 0.74; 95% CI, 0.60–0.91). Elseviers and colleagues[10] examined 987 institutions with a mean of 96.8 (±47.4) beds per institution and found that larger nursing homes had a lower average consumption of drugs per patient. To estimate the effect of nursing home size, Chiang and associates[6] divided their sample into large nursing homes and small nursing homes based on the mean number of beds per nursing home (140). They found large nursing home size was associated with lower number of total medications.

Other facility characteristics
Dwyer and colleagues[8] showed that patients in for-profit nursing homes had a lower prevalence of polypharmacy than patients in not-for-profit nursing homes (OR, 0.84; 95% CI, 0.75–0.95) on multivariate analyses. Wayne and associates[13] showed no significant differences in medication prescription by level of care (intermediate care facility vs skilled nursing facility).

Nursing home length of stay
Studies of nursing home length of stay (LOS) and polypharmacy have had mixed results. Dwyer and colleagues[8] broke down LOS since admission to less than 3 months, 3 to more than 6 months, 6 months to less than 1 year, 1 to more 3 years, 3 to fewer than 5 years, and 5 years or longer. Multivariate analyses showed that compared with those with a LOS of less than 3 months (reference), residents with LOS of 3 to less than 6 months were significantly more likely to receive polypharmacy (OR, 1.25; 95% CI, 1.04–1.50), whereas those with a LOS 5 years or longer were significantly less likely to receive polypharmacy (OR, 0.68; 95% CI, 0.56–0.82). Arinzon and co-wrkers[39] performed a cross-sectional study in 324 patients in an Israeli nursing home between 2001 and 2002. They found no difference in the overall number of drugs between the newly admitted patients versus institutionalized patients (defined as LOS ≥3 months). Wayne and associates[13] found a significant increase in the total number of medications prescribed per patient with LOS, with a mean of 4.7 medications at admission to the nursing home compared with a mean of

6.2 medications after 3 months. Chen and colleagues[7] found no differences in mean total number of medications at 4 data collection points: On admission, 6 months before death, 3 months before death, and at death.

Insurance and place of residence before nursing home

Studies looking at polypharmacy and insurance or place of residence before nursing home placement have demonstrated mixed results. Dwyer and associates[8] studied the primary payment sources of Medicaid, out-of-pocket/private, Medicare, unknown, and other insurance. Multivariate analyses showed that patients whose primary payment source was out-of-pocket/private were less likely to receive polypharmacy (OR, 0.66; 95% CI, 0.58–0.75) compared with Medicaid and Medicare patients. Koopmans and associates[40] found that patients who had been living at home before admission were prescribed fewer drugs than those who were admitted from a residential home or hospital (4.1, 6.3, and 6.1, respectively). In contrast, Balogun and colleagues[12] found no difference in the number of medications prescribed when comparing patients admitted to the nursing homes from different sources (acute hospitals, other nursing homes, acute rehabilitation centers, home, and assisted living facilities).

DISCUSSION

This article provides a comprehensive review of factors associated with polypharmacy in nursing homes. Our review has some limitations. First, we included studies beginning in 1990, and may have excluded significant, earlier studies. We used MEDLINE as our primary search engine; thus, studies identifiable only with other search engines may not have been included. However, we did search for related and cited papers in our search strategy, reducing the likelihood of missing important studies. Only English-language articles were included. For this review, we defined polypharmacy as the use of high number of medications. Others have defined polypharmacy as use of medications that are not indicated or unnecessary.

We found that age was significantly associated with number of medications in approximately half the studies reviewed. There are several possible explanations for an association between age and number of medications among nursing home patients. One reason may be the healthy survival effect, with the "oldest old" being healthier and therefore taking fewer medications. Other explanations may be that physicians are more careful in their prescribing to the oldest old; the "young old" may need and/or request more medications, or the young old are more likely to be admitted to nursing homes from acute care settings where they receive complex medication regimens (eg, recovery from surgery, infections).

The studies of gender and polypharmacy found mixed results. Some studies showed no association, whereas others found that women take more medications. Only 1 study found that men take more medications. One possible reason for these discrepancies is that some of these studies looked at total medications, whereas others looked at scheduled medications.

Most studies found that cognitive impairment and dementia were associated with decreased polypharmacy. The inverse relationship between cognitive status and drug use has not been well investigated, but there are several possible explanations. One possible explanation may be that cognitively impaired patients who enter nursing homes have less comorbidity compared with patients with normal cognitive function. The cognitively impaired/demented patient may become a nursing home resident not because of multiple comorbidities, but because of their mental status. Dementia may reduce mental stress and thus be protective against possible stress-contributing conditions such as hypertension and heart diseases. Physicians may tend to underdiagnose conditions and underprescribe medications to these patients because this population may not be able to communicate their complaints well. Another possible explanation is that physicians may be appropriately reducing medications owing to recognition of advanced dementia and diminishing medication benefit. Patients may also have difficulty taking and swallowing medications. One of the challenges of treating dementia is that it is a chronic, progressive disease; the goals of care change with each stage. Further studies are needed to define appropriate medication use in each stage of dementia according to the goals of care. To date, there have been few studies to define the role of medications in dementia or the impact of medication discontinuation in persons with end-stage dementia.[35] Treatment guidelines provided little direction on how to determine benefit, how long to treat, and under what conditions to discontinue these medications.

It was not surprising that number of medications was linked to a greater number of comorbidities. It was also not surprising that patients with more prescribers were given more medications. The acuity of patients requiring multiple prescribers is likely higher than patients cared for by only 1 prescriber. However, it is also possible that this relationship may be partly owing to lack of communication between prescribers. Similarly, we found that more medications were used if more than 1 pharmacy was involved. It may be difficult to manage a patient's profile if medications are supplied by more than 1 pharmacy.

Larger nursing homes seemed to have less polypharmacy. Large facilities are more likely to have greater resources, which may include specialty physicians, nurse practitioners, and other specialty clinicians. They are also more likely to have an in-house pharmacist consultant who conducts regular reviews of patients' drug regimens.

SUMMARY

The prevalence of polypharmacy is very high in the nursing home setting. In this comprehensive review, we describe the many demographic, functional status, chronic disease, and healthcare financing factors associated with polypharmacy in nursing home patients. Recognition of the factors associated with polypharmacy is the first step for practitioners. A quality improvement intervention study previously conducted by the authors of this paper demonstrated that polypharmacy can be reduced in the nursing setting as a result of systematic review of medications by physicians.[41]

DISCLOSURE

This research was supported by The John A. Hartford Foundation Center of Excellence in Geriatrics, University of Hawaii; the funding source had no role in the analysis and preparation of this paper. Dr Bell received compensation for participation in Aloha Care, a local insurance company Pharmacy and Therapeutics committee. Drs Tamura, Inaba and Masaki have no conflicts to declare.

REFERENCES

1. inkers F, Maring JG, Boersma F, et al. A study of medication reviews to identify drug-related problems of polypharmacy patients in the Dutch nursing home setting. J Clin Pharm Ther 2007;32:469–76.
2. Lau DT, Kasper JD, Potter DE, et al. Potentially inappropriate medication prescriptions among elderly nursing home residents: their scope and associated resident and facility characteristics. Health Serv Res 2004;39:1257–76.
3. Ostrom JR, Hammarlund ER, Christensen DB, et al. Medication usage in an elderly population. Med Care 1985;23:157–64.

4. Gupta S, Rappaport HM, Bennett LT. Polypharmacy among nursing home geriatric Medicaid recipients. Ann Pharmacother 1996;30:946–50.
5. Bergman A, Olsson J, Carlsten A, et al. Evaluation of the quality of drug therapy among elderly patients in nursing homes. Scand J Prim Health Care 2007;25:9–14.
6. Chiang L, Hirsch SH, Reuben DB. Predictors of medication prescription in nursing homes. J Am Med Dir Assoc 2000;1:97–102.
7. Chen IC, Liu ML, Twu FC, et al. Use of medication by nursing home residents nearing end of life: a preliminary report. J Nurs Res 2010;18:199–205.
8. Dwyer LL, Han B, Woodwell DA, et al. Polypharmacy in nursing home residents in the United States: results of the 2004 National Nursing Home Survey. Am J Geriatr Pharmacother 2010;8:63–72.
9. Olsson J, Bergman A, Carlsten A, et al. Quality of drug prescribing in elderly people in nursing homes and special care units for dementia: a cross-sectional computerized pharmacy register analysis. Clin Drug Investig 2010;30:289–300.
10. Elseviers MM, Vander Stichele RR, Van Bortel L. Drug utilization in Belgian nursing homes: impact of residents' and institutional characteristics. Pharmacoepidemiol Drug Saf 2010;19:1041–8.
11. Beers MH, Ouslander JG, Fingold SF, et al. Inappropriate medication prescribing in skilled-nursing facilities. Ann Intern Med 1992;117:684–9.
12. Balogun S PM, Evans J. Potentially inappropriate medications in nursing homes: sources and correlates. Internet Journal of Geriatrics and Gerontology 2005;2(2).
13. Wayne SJ, Rhyne RL, Stratton M. Longitudinal prescribing patterns in a nursing home population. J Am Geriatr Soc 1992;40:53–6.
14. Hanlon JT, Wang X, Good CB, et al. Racial differences in medication use among older, long-stay Veterans Affairs nursing home care unit patients. Consult Pharm 2009;24: 439–46.
15. Welch HG, Walsh JS, Larson EB. The cost of institutional care in Alzheimer's disease: nursing home and hospital use in a prospective cohort. J Am Geriatr Soc 1992;40: 221–4.
16. Magaziner J, German P, Zimmerman SI, et al. The prevalence of dementia in a statewide sample of new nursing home admissions aged 65 and older: diagnosis by expert panel. Epidemiology of Dementia in Nursing Homes Research Group. Gerontologist 2000;40:663–72.
17. Tjia J, Rothman MR, Kiely DK, et al. Daily medication use in nursing home residents with advanced dementia. J Am Geriatr Soc 2010;58:880–8.
18. Dhall J, Larrat EP, Lapane KL. Use of potentially inappropriate drugs in nursing homes. Pharmacotherapy 2002;22:88–96.
19. Landi F, Gambassi G, Lapane KL, et al. Comorbidity and drug use in cognitively impaired elderly living in long-term care. Dement Geriatr Cogn Disord 1998;9:347–56.
20. Katz S, Ford AB, Moskowitz RW, et al. Studies of Illness in the Aged. The Index of Adl: A Standardized Measure of Biological and Psychosocial Function. JAMA 1963;185: 914–9.
21. Hosia-Randell HM, Muurinen SM, Pitkala KH. Exposure to potentially inappropriate drugs and drug-drug interactions in elderly nursing home residents in Helsinki, Finland: a cross-sectional study. Drugs Aging 2008;25:683–92.
22. Nygaard HA, Naik M, Ruths S, Straand J. Nursing-home residents and their drug use: a comparison between mentally intact and mentally impaired residents. The Bergen district nursing home (BEDNURS) study. Eur J Clin Pharmacol 2003;59:463–9.
23. Folstein MF, Folstein SE, McHugh PR. "Mini-mental state". A practical method for grading the cognitive state of patients for the clinician. J Psychiatr Res 1975;12: 189–98.

24. Holmes HM, Sachs GA, Shega JW, et al. Integrating palliative medicine into the care of persons with advanced dementia: identifying appropriate medication use. J Am Geriatr Soc 2008;56:1306–11.

25. Briesacher BA, Limcangco MR, Simoni-Wastila L, et al. The quality of antipsychotic drug prescribing in nursing homes. Arch Intern Med 2005;165:1280–5.

26. Ballard CG, Thomas A, Fossey J, et al. A 3-month, randomized, placebo-controlled, neuroleptic discontinuation study in 100 people with dementia: the neuropsychiatric inventory median cutoff is a predictor of clinical outcome. J Clin Psychiatry 2004;65: 114–9.

27. Cohen-Mansfield J, Lipson S, Werner P, et al. Withdrawal of haloperidol, thioridazine, and lorazepam in the nursing home: a controlled, double-blind study. Arch Intern Med 1999;159:1733–40.

28. Mitchell SL, Kiely DK, Hamel MB. Dying with advanced dementia in the nursing home. Arch Intern Med 2004;164:321–6.

29. Blass DM, Black BS, Phillips H, et al. Medication use in nursing home residents with advanced dementia. Int J Geriatr Psychiatry 2008;23:490–6.

30. Bridges-Parlet S, Knopman D, Steffes S. Withdrawal of neuroleptic medications from institutionalized dementia patients: results of a double-blind, baseline-treatment-controlled pilot study. J Geriatr Psychiatry Neurol 1997;10:119–26.

31. Ruths S, Straand J, Nygaard HA, et al. Effect of antipsychotic withdrawal on behavior and sleep/wake activity in nursing home residents with dementia: a randomized, placebo-controlled, double-blinded study. The Bergen District Nursing Home Study. J Am Geriatr Soc 2004;52:1737–43.

32. van Reekum R, Clarke D, Conn D, et al. A randomized, placebo-controlled trial of the discontinuation of long-term antipsychotics in dementia. Int Psychogeriatr 2002;14: 197–210.

33. Gruber-Baldini AL, Stuart B, Zuckerman IH, et al. Treatment of dementia in community-dwelling and institutionalized medicare beneficiaries. J Am Geriatr Soc 2007;55: 1508–16.

34. Herrmann N, Gill SS, Bell CM, et al. A population-based study of cholinesterase inhibitor use for dementia. J Am Geriatr Soc 2007;55:1517–23.

35. Weschules DJ, Maxwell TL, Shega JW. Acetylcholinesterase inhibitor and N-methyl-D-aspartic acid receptor antagonist use among hospice enrollees with a primary diagnosis of dementia. J Palliat Med 2008;11:738–45.

36. Parsons C, Briesacher BA, Givens JL, et al. Cholinesterase inhibitor and memantine use in newly admitted nursing home residents with dementia. J Am Geriatr Soc 2011;59:1253–9.

37. Burrows AB, Morris JN, Simon SE, et al. Development of a minimum data set-based depression rating scale for use in nursing homes. Age Ageing 2000;29:165–72.

38. Suominen M, Muurinen S, Routasalo P, et al. Malnutrition and associated factors among aged residents in all nursing homes in Helsinki. Eur J Clin Nutr 2005;59: 578–83.

39. Arinzon Z, Peisakh A, Zuta A, et al. Drug use in a geriatric long-term care setting: comparison between newly admitted and institutionalised patients. Drugs Aging 2006;23:157–65.

40. Koopmans RT, van der Borgh JP, Bor JH, et al. Increase in drug use after admission to Dutch nursing homes. Pharm World Sci 2003;25:30–4.

41. Tamura BK, Bell CL, Lubimir K, et al. Physician intervention for medication reduction in a nursing home: the polypharmacy outcomes project. J Am Med Dir Assoc 2011;12:326–30.

Outcomes of Polypharmacy in Nursing Home Residents

Bruce K. Tamura, MD*, Christina L. Bell, MD, MS,
Michiko Inaba, MD, PhD, Kamal H. Masaki, MD

KEYWORDS

- Long-term care • Polypharmacy • Nursing home
- Outcomes

Are there significant adverse outcomes of polypharmacy in nursing home patients? Polypharmacy is of special concern in the elderly because they have higher susceptibility to side effects and develop toxicity to certain drugs more easily than young people.[1] The authors of this review previously completed a quality improvement intervention study, which demonstrated reduced polypharmacy in a nursing home as a result of systematic medication review by geriatricians and geriatric medicine fellows.[2] There are few systematic reviews of outcomes of polypharmacy in long-term care. This summary of the literature is targeted toward clinicians practicing in long-term care.

METHODS

We conducted a MEDLINE search using such words as polypharmacy, medication, nursing home, long-term care, adverse effects, mortality, death, hospitalization, fracture, falls, and cost. We reviewed only English-language articles starting from 1990. We included primarily original articles specific to nursing homes, and excluded nursing home articles that included home-bound patients, outpatients, assisted living, or hospital settings. There are many definitions of polypharmacy in the literature, including number of medications or use of inappropriate medications. In this review, we defined polypharmacy as a high number of medications, but not inappropriate medications. We extracted the data from articles systematically using standardized tables. Data were sorted by size of study and outcomes of polypharmacy.

RESULTS

Potentially Inappropriate Drugs

Potentially inappropriate drugs can be defined as those in which the risk of adverse events from the drug outweighs the clinical benefits, and in particular, where there is a safer and more effective alternative **(Table 1)**.[3] Potentially inappropriate drugs are

Department of Geriatric Medicine, The John A. Hartford Center of Excellence in Geriatrics, 347 North Kuakini Street, HPM-9, Honolulu, HI 96817, USA
* Corresponding author.
E-mail address: bktamura@hotmail.com

Clin Geriatr Med 28 (2012) 217–236
doi:10.1016/j.cger.2012.01.005
0749-0690/12/$ – see front matter © 2012 Elsevier Inc. All rights reserved.

Table 1
Potentially Inappropriate Drugs (PID) as outcomes associated with polypharmacy in nursing home patient populations

Author and Year	Study Population, Setting, Year and Data Source	Results
Dhall[7] 2002	n = 44,562 new patients in NHs in 5 states using 1995–1996 MDS data	Higher number of drugs associated with higher likelihood of PID: 4–5 meds (OR, 1.7; 95% CI, 1.6–1.9); 6–8 meds (OR, 2.4; 95% CI, 2.2–2.6); ≥9 meds (OR, 3.5; 95% CI, 3.2–3.8); reference, using 1–3 meds
Williams[9] 1995	n = 21,884 patients in NHs in 2 states using 1991 MDS data	Higher number of drugs associated with higher likelihood of PID: 4–6 meds (OR, 2.18); ≥7 meds (OR, 3.81); reference, ≤3 meds; P<.05
Lau[1] 2004	n = 3,372 NHs patients, nationally representative sample of 1.6 million patients in 1996 database[a]	Higher number of drugs associated with higher likelihood of PID: <5 meds (OR, 0.23; 95% CI, 0.19–0.29); 5 to<9 meds (OR, 0.46; 95% CI, 0.37–0.56); using ≥9 meds as reference, P<.001
Rancourt[11] 2004	n = 2633 patients in Quebec NHs, cross-sectional chart review in 1995–1996	Higher number of drugs associated with higher likelihood of PID: OR, 1.36 (95% CI, 1.32–1.41) for increase in increment of 1 drug
Stafford[14] 2011	n = 2345 patients in Australian NHs using 2006–2007 pharmacist database	Polypharmacy (≥6 meds) associated with higher likelihood of PID: OR, 2.07 (95% CI, 1.53–2.80); P<.001
Hosia-Randell[16] 2008	n = 1987 patients in Finland NHs in 2003 using chart review	Among patients with PIDs, 56% were on ≥9 meds/d compared with patients without PIDs with 35.7% on ≥9 meds/day (95% CI, 0.158–0.248); P<.001
Ruggiero[6] 2010	n = 1716 patients in Italy NHs, multicenter prospective 1-year study in 2004	Higher number of drugs (>5) associated with higher likelihood of PID (P<.0001)
Niwata[17] 2006	n = 1669 patients in Japan NHs, cross-sectional chart review in 2002	Higher number of drugs associated with higher likelihood of PID: OR, 1.14 (95% CI, 1.08–1.21) for each increase in med number; correlation coefficient, 0.27 (P<.0001)
Perri[18] 2005	n = 1117 patients in Georgia NHs using 2002 Medicaid data and chart review	Higher number of drugs associated with higher likelihood of PID: OR, 1.13 (95% CI, 1.10–1.17) for each increase in med number (P<.001)

Nygaard[19] 2003	n = 1042 patients in 15 Norwegian NHs using 1996–1997 Pharmacy data	PID weakly correlated with total number of drugs used ($r = 0.33$; $P < .001$)
Mamun[20] 2004	n = 454 patients in 3 Singapore NHs, data collected by chart review	Polypharmacy (≥5 meds) associated with PID ($P < .001$)
Chiang[22] 2000	n = 414 patients at 20 NHs in 3 states, data collected by chart review	Higher number of drugs only significant predictor of PID ($P < .001$)
Gill[23] 2001	n = 355 patients in 1 London Ontario NH in 1999 using chart review	Patients with PID a mean of 8.49 meds; patients with no PID a mean of 6.59 meds ($P < .001$)
Balogun[27] 2005	n = 175 patients in 2 Virginia NHs in 2002, cross-sectional admission data set	Of patients with polypharmacy (≥12 meds), 51.4% with PID and 48.6% with no PID; of patients with PID, 64.3% had polypharmacy, 35.7% did not ($P < .001$ for both analyses)

Abbreviations: CI, confidence interval; NH, nursing home; OR, odds ratio.
[a] Medical expenditure panel survey NH component.

a major determinant of adverse drug events (ADEs)[4] and have been associated with an increased risk of hospitalization or death.[1,5,6] There have been many studies demonstrating that polypharmacy was associated with increased likelihood of being prescribed a potentially inappropriate drug.

Dhall and colleageus[7] performed a review of the Minimum Data Set (MDS) for 44,562 new patients in nursing homes in 5 states. Inappropriate drugs were classified based on the Beers criteria.[8] As the number of prescribed drugs increased, the likelihood of receiving inappropriate drugs increased. Patients taking 9 or more drugs were about 4 times as likely as those taking 1 to 3 drugs to be taking a potentially inappropriate drug, after controlling for other factors. Williams and Betley[9] reviewed 1991 MDS data of 21,884 patients in 2 states, to study 10 of the 30 inappropriate medications identified by Beers and associates.[10] Multivariate models showed a generally linear relationship between the total number of standing medications and the likelihood of receiving an inappropriate medication. The odds of receiving at least 1 inappropriate medication was significantly higher among patients receiving 4 to 6 or 7 or more standing medications (odds ratio [OR], 2.18; 95% confidence interval [CI], 1.90–2.50; and OR, 3.81, 95% CI, 3.30–4.40, respectively), compared with patients receiving 0 to 3 standing medications.

Lau and colleagues[1] examined 3372 patients in nursing homes in 1996, representative of 1.6 million nursing home patients in the United States. Patients were considered to have a potentially inappropriate drug exposure if any of the following conditions were met: (1) Medication names matched "inappropriate drug choice" in Beers criteria; (2) strengths and average dosages of medications matched those defined as "excessive dosage" in Beers criteria; or (3) patients had active diagnoses and took medications that matched any of the "drug–disease interactions" in Beers criteria.[8,10] Patients taking fewer than 5 drugs monthly were only one quarter as likely, and those taking 5 to 9 drugs only half as likely, to have a potentially inappropriate drug compared with those taking 9 or more medications.

Rancourt and associates[11] performed a cross-sectional chart review of 2633 patients in long-term care facilities in Quebec. They created a list of 111 explicit criteria and potentially inappropriate prescriptions were categorized as: (1) Potentially inappropriate medications, (2) potentially inappropriate duration, (3) potentially inappropriate dosage, and (4) potentially inappropriate drug–drug interactions (DDIs). Multivariate analysis showed the risk of a potentially inappropriate prescription increased significantly as the number of drugs prescribed increased. Stafford and colleagues used the Beers criteria[8,10,12] and the McLeod criteria[13] for determining inappropriate medication prescribing.[14] Multivariate analysis showed the number of medications (≥6 medications vs 0–5 medications) predicted inappropriate prescribing using both criteria.

Hosia-Randell and associates used the updated Beers criteria[15] to identify potentially inappropriate drug use independent of diagnoses or conditions,[16] and found that patients taking potentially inappropriate drugs were more likely to use 9 or more drugs per day. Ruggiero and co-workers[6] used the updated Beers criteria[15] and showed that number of drugs was associated with a high likelihood of using a potentially inappropriate drug. Niwata and colleagues[17] used the updated Beers criteria[15] to identify potentially inappropriate medications, and found that the number of medications used per day increased the risk of inappropriate medication use. Perri and colleagues[18] used the Beers criteria[8] in their review of patients' chart to identify inappropriate medication use, which was defined as any medication on the Beers list. Patients taking a greater number of medications were more likely to receive a potentially inappropriate drug. Nygaard and associates[19] used the Beers criteria[8] to define inappropriate drug use, which was weakly but significantly correlated with the total number of drugs used. Mamun and co-workers[20] used the Beers criteria[8] to determine appropriateness of medications. Medications not specified by the Beers criteria were further analyzed on the basis of 8 drug related problem categories developed by Strand and co-wrokers.[21] They found an association between polypharmacy (≥5 medications) and inappropriate medication use. Chiang and colleagues[22] classified medications as inappropriate based on the Beers criteria,[12] and found that higher number of total medications was the only significant predictor of higher use of inappropriate medications.

Gill and associates[23] determined inappropriate prescribing using the Improving Prescribing in the Elderly Tool,[24] Charlson comorbidity index,[25] and the MDS.[26] Patients with potentially inappropriate prescriptions were taking a larger number of medications. Balogun and co-workers[27] used the updated Beers criteria[15] to define potentially inappropriate medications. Overall number of medications used was associated with potentially inappropriate medications prescribed, with 64% of patients on a potentially inappropriate medication also taking 12 or more medications.

ADEs and DDIs

Older patients are at greater risk for ADEs because they often have complex drug regimens and because of age-related changes in drug pharmacokinetics and pharmacodynamics.[28] ADEs can include preventable and unavoidable medication-related events that lead to potentially negative patient outcomes.[29–31] ADEs can result from medication errors or adverse drug reactions (ADRs).[30–33] The majority of the studies we reviewed showed that polypharmacy was associated with increased likelihood of having an ADE and/or a DDI **(Table 2)**.

Ruths and associates[34] used a 4-member physician/pharmacist panel to perform a comprehensive medication review and compile a list of significant medication problems. One single problem could involve several drugs and 1 single prescription might cause several problems. The panel identified 2445 drug-related problems in 1036 patients. Examples of drug-related problems included risk for ADR, DDI, dosage of medication too high, and excessive treatment duration. The number of problems identified was significantly associated with number of drugs used per patient. Field and colleagues[32] defined ADEs as injuries resulting from use of a drug. Preventable ADEs were those that resulted from medication error in prescribing, dispensing, administering, or monitoring. ADRs were synonymous with nonpreventable ADEs in which no error was involved. As the number of regularly scheduled medications increased, the odds of having an ADE increased. Taking 7 to 8 and 9 or more regularly scheduled medications were independently associated with having a preventable ADE. Nguyen and colleagues[31] identified potential ADRs through voluntary ADR reporting by health care professionals and through monitoring trigger events. Trigger events included emergency room visits, admission to acute care, death, premature discontinuation of a medication, initiation of a medication typically used for treatment of a hypersensitivity reaction, initiation of a medication to treat acute confusional states, deterioration of underlying disease, rash or other physical change, falls, and behavioral/cognitive changes. Two investigators blinded to the presence of polypharmacy independently applied the Naranjo ADR probability scale.[35–37] Controlling for age and gender, subjects using 9 or more scheduled medications were 2.33 times more likely than controls to experience an ADR. Cooper[38] used the technique described by Naranjo[37] to report probable ADRs, and found that the only difference between the groups with and without ADRs was the mean number of drugs per patient (7.8 ± 2.6 vs 3.3 ± 1.3, respectively). Gerety and associates[39] applied the algorithm described by Naranjo[37] to classify ADEs

Table 2
Adverse Drug Events (ADE) and Drug–Drug Interactions (DDI) as outcomes associated with polypharmacy in nursing home patient populations

Author and Year	Study Population, Setting, Year and Data Source	Results
ADE		
Ruths[34] 2003	n = 1354 patients in Norway NHs in 1997 using cross-sectional chart review	Higher number of drugs associated with higher number of drug-related problems (r = 0.14; P< .0001)
Field[32] 2001	n = 410 patients in 18 Massachusetts NHs, 1997 case-control chart review study nested in 12-month prospective study of ADEs	Higher number of drugs associated with higher likelihood of ADR: 5–6 meds (OR, 2.0; 95% CI, 1.2–3.2), 7–8 meds (OR, 2.8; 95% CI, 1.7–4.7); ≥9 meds (OR, 3.3; 95% CI, 1.9–5.6), using <5 meds as reference
Field[32] 2001	n = 410 patients in 18 Massachusetts NHs, 1997 case-control chart review study nested in 12-month prospective study of ADEs	Higher number of drugs associated with higher likelihood of preventable ADR[a]: 5–6 meds (OR, 1.7; 95% CI, 0.83–3.5); 7–8 meds (OR, 3.2; 95% CI, 1.4–6.9); ≥9 meds (OR, 2.9; 95% CI, 1.3–6.8); using <5 meds as reference
Nguyen[31] 2006	n = 335 patients (excluded hospice, respite, and rehabilitation) in 1 California SNF in 1998 using chart review	Higher number of drugs (≥9 meds) associated with higher likelihood of ADR: OR, 2.33 (95% CI, 1.54–3.52); using <9 meds as reference (P< .001)
Cooper[38] 1996	n = 332 patients in Georgia NHs, monthly drug review	Patients with a probable ADR were on a mean of 7.8 ± 2.6 vs 3.3 ± 1.3 drugs for those with no ADR (P< .001)
Gerety[39] 1993	n = 175 new patients in 1 VA NH in 1988–1989 using chart review	Higher number of drugs not associated with number of ADR (r = 0.24; P = .09)
Gerety[39] 1993	n = 175 new patients in 1 VA NH in 1988–1989 using chart review	Higher number of drugs associated with number of ADWE (r = 0.29); multiple linear regression (P = .005); number of meds had borderline association with at ≥1 ADWE (P = .05 [correlation]; P = .005 [linear regression]; P = .08 [logistic regression])

DDI		
Hosia-Randell[16] 2008	n = 1987 patients in Finland NHs in 2003 using chart review	Among patients with potential for class D DDIs, 58.3% were on ≥9 meds/day, compared with 42.0% patients with no potential for class D DDIs (95%CI, −0.051 to −0.011; P = .002)
Liao[40] 2008	n = 323 patients in Taiwan NHs in 2006 using chart review	Higher number of meds associated with higher likelihood of DDI: ≥9 meds (OR, 11.4; 95% CI, 2.7–46.2), using 1–2 meds as reference (P = .001)

Abbreviations: ADR, adverse drug reaction; ADWE, adverse drug withdrawal events.

[a] A preventable ADE is from an error (prescribing, dispensing, administering or monitoring) and preventable by any means currently available.

related to drug administration, and devised a similar algorithm to determine the probability that clinical adverse events were related to drug discontinuation, namely, adverse drug withdrawal events (ADWEs). They found no association between number of medications and ADEs. However, number of medications had a significant independent association with ADWE frequency in multivariate models. Patients who experienced at least 1 ADWE took more medications. Hosia-Randell and co-workers[16] used the Swedish, Finnish, Interaction X-referencing medical interaction database that includes information on more than 6200 DDIs.[16] Patients exposed to potential DDIs were more likely to be taking 9 or more drugs per day. This included class D interactions, which are clinically significant, and suggest that the combination should be avoided. Liao and colleagues[40] used the DDI Database Information System constructed by the Department of Health, Executive Yuan, Taiwan, to match recorded medications, and found that the likelihood of DDIs was higher with a greater number of medications.

Falls and Fractures

Injury is the fifth leading cause of death in older adults, and most of these fatal injuries are related to falls **(Table 3)**.[41] Falls account for over 80% of injury-related hospital admissions in people older than 65 years.[41] Between 10% and 25% of nursing home falls result in fractures or hospital admissions.[42] Studies about the association between polypharmacy and falls/fractures have had mixed results.

Baranzini and co-workers[43] defined a fall as a sudden and unintentional change of position, with or without loss of consciousness, causing the victim to land on the ground.[44] Fall-related injuries included abrasions, cuts, fractures, dislocations, loss of consciousness, and emergency department visits. The prevalence of injuries was not found to be related to number of medications. Taking an anti-arrhythmic or anti-Parkinson drug as part of a regimen of 7 or more medications was associated with a 3-fold increased risk of reporting a fall-related injury. Yip and Cumming[45] defined falls as all events for which the staff filed an incident report for a "fall." Patients who fell at least once during the study period constituted the case group, and the control group comprised those who did not fall during the same period. Being prescribed 4 or more drugs was not associated with increased falls. Lipsitz and associates[46] reviewed charts of recurrent fallers and nonfallers in 2 Massachusetts nursing homes, and found that 75% of patients taking 7 or more medications fell, compared with 60% of those taking 4 to 6 medications, and 40% of those taking 1 to 3 medications. Compared with nonfallers, fallers took on average 1 more medication. Kerman and Mulvihill[47] found that after controlling for ambulatory status, fallers were taking an average of 1.05 more drugs than controls.

Chen and associates performed 2 studies of radiographically confirmed fractures and number of medications.[48,49] In the 2-year follow-up period, use of 7 or more medications was associated with higher fracture rate. However, when the follow-up period was extended to 4 years, they found that use of 7 or more medications was not associated with increased hip fractures.

Hospitalization and Mortality

Most of the studies we reviewed found that increasing number of medications was associated with a higher likelihood of hospitalization **(Table 4)**. Dedhiya and colleagues[50] used a logistic regression model controlling for demographic and clinical characteristics, and showed that the likelihood of hospitalization increased significantly with an increase in number of medications. Mathew and co-workers[51] studied patients with chronic kidney disease who were admitted for potentially avoidable

Table 3
Falls and fractures as outcomes associated with polypharmacy in Nursing Home (NH) patient populations

Author and Year	Study Population, Setting, Year and Data Source	Results
Falls		
Baranzini[43] 2009	n = 221 patients in 1 Italy NH in 2004–2007 using chart review	Polypharmacy (≥7 meds) was not associated with fall-related injuries ($P = .50$); polypharmacy (≥7 meds) + (antiarrhythmic med or anti-Parkinson med, interaction term) associated with fall-related injuries (OR, 4.4; 95% CI, 1.21–15.36; $P = .024$)
Yip[45] 1994	n = 71 patients in 1 Australian NH in 1990–1991 using chart review	Number of prescribed drugs (≥4 meds) was not significantly associated with falls: Crude RR, 1.03 (95% CI, 0.75–1.42)
Lipsitz[46] 1991	n = 70 recurrent fallers and 56 nonfallers in 2 Massachusetts NHs in 1986–1989 using chart review	15/20 (75%) of patients on ≥7 meds fell; 37/62 (60%) of patients on 4–6 meds fell; 18/44 (41%) of patients on 1–3 meds fell ($P = .002$)
Kerman[47] 1990	n = 57 patients in 1 NY NH in 1987–1988 using chart review	Fallers had a mean of 5.37 meds; nonfallers had a mean of 4.32 meds ($P<.001$)
Fractures		
Chen[49] 2008	n = 2005 patients in Australia NHs in 1999–2003 with 2-year fracture follow up	Polypharmacy (≥7 meds) was significantly associated with fractures: HR, 1.30 (95% CI, 1.04–1.62), using 0–6 meds as reference ($P = .02$)
Chen[48] 2009	n = 1894 patients in 52 Australia NHs + 30 ICF in 1999–2003, with 4-year fracture follow-up	Polypharmacy (≥7 meds) was not significantly associated with hip fractures: HR, 0.95 (95% CI, 0.72–1.26), using 0–6 meds as reference ($P = .72$)

Abbreviations: CI, confidence interval; HR, hazard ratio; ICF, intermediate care facility.

hospitalizations, namely, ambulatory care sensitive hospitalizations.[52] Using multivariate logistic regression, they found that patients on more than 12 medications were more likely to be hospitalized compared with those on 12 or fewer medications. Intrator and associates[53] studied 2080 patients in 1993 using MDS data. Use of more than 6 medications per week was associated with hospitalization. Tang and colleagues[54] performed a cross-sectional MDS database study of 1820 Chinese nursing home patients in 2001, and found that polypharmacy (≥7 medications) was associated with increased hospitalization. Ruggiero and associates[6] reported that patients admitted to the hospital were taking more drugs compared with patients not admitted to the hospital (5.85 ± 3.16 vs 5.02 ± 2.81, respectively). Cherubini and co-workers[55] performed an observational, multicenter, prospective 1-year cohort study of 1683 long-term nursing home residents in 31 nursing homes in Italy in 2004. Polypharmacy

Table 4
Hospitalization and mortality as outcomes associated with polypharmacy in nursing home patient populations

Author and Year	Study Population, Setting, Year, and Data Source	Results
Hospitalization		
Dedhiya[50] 2010	n = 7594 NH patients in Indiana using 2002 Medicaid claims data	Higher number of drugs (per year) associated with higher likelihood of hospitalization: 11–15 meds, OR, 1.28 (95% CI, 1.04-1.57; P = .018); 16–20 meds, OR, 1.46 (95% CI, 1.19-1.81; $P<$.001); >20 meds, OR, 1.63 (95% CI, 1.32–2.02; $P<$.001); reference, using 1–10 meds
Mathew[51] 2011	n = 5449 NH patients in NY with chronic kidney disease and hospitalized in 2007, using MDS and NH datasets	Higher number of drugs (>12 meds) significantly associated with higher likelihood of hospitalization: OR, 1.30 (95% CI, 1.15–1.47)
Intrator[53] 1999	n = 2080 patients in 10 states in 1993, using MDS data	Receiving >6 medications per week was associated with higher likelihood of hospitalization (OR, 1.27; CI, 0.95–1.72)
Tang[54] 2010	n = 1820 patients in Hong Kong, cross-sectional, using MDS data	Polypharmacy (≥7 medications) was associated with a greater likelihood of hospitalization (P = .016)
Ruggiero[6] 2010	n = 1716 patients in Italy NHs, multicenter prospective 1-year study in 2004	Patients who were hospitalized were on more meds than nonhospitalized patients, mean 5.85 ± 3.16 meds vs 5.02 ± 2.81 meds (P = .0004)
Cherubini[55] 2011	n = 1683 patients in Italy NHs in 2004, observational, prospective cohort over 1 year	Polypharmacy (>5 meds) was a risk factor for hospitalization (P = .0028)
Hui[56] 2000	n = 606 patients in 5 NHs in Hong Kong	Polypharmacy (≥5 meds) was a risk factor for hospitalization (P = .03)
Ouslander[57] 2010	n = 377 patients in Georgia NHs in 2005 using Medicare data	No significant difference in hospitalization rates with polypharmacy: NHs with highest rates of hospitalization had 64% of patients with polypharmacy (≥9 meds); NHs with lowest rates of hospitalization had 62% of patients with polypharmacy
Cooper[58] 1999	n = 332 patients in Georgia SNFs, 4-year prospective observational study	Patients with probable ADR hospitalization were on higher mean number of meds 7.9 ± 2.6 meds vs patients with no ADRs 3.3 ± 1.3 meds ($P<$.001)

Mortality

Dedhiya[50] 2010	n = 7594 NH patients in Indiana using 2002 Medicaid claims data	Higher number of drugs (per year) associated with decreased likelihood of mortality: 11–15 meds, OR, 0.75 (95% CI, 0.66–0.86); 16–20 meds, OR, 0.76 (95% CI, 0.66–0.88); >20 meds, OR, 0.75 (95% CI, 0.65–0.87); using 1–10 meds as reference ($P<.001$)
Intrator[53] 1999	n = 2080 patients in 10 states in 1993, using MDS data	Receiving >6 medications per week was not significantly associated with higher likelihood of death (OR, 1.06; 95% CI, 0.70–1.60)
Leung[59] 1997	n = 411 patients in Taiwan NHs in 1992, baseline survey with 3-year follow-up for mortality	Higher number of drugs not significantly associated with likelihood of mortality: 1–2 meds, OR, 1.04 (95% CI, 0.63–1.72); ≥3 meds, OR, 0.90 (95% CI, 0.43–1.86); using 0 medications as reference

Abbreviations: ADR, adverse drug reaction; CI, confidence interval; MDS, Minimum Data Set; NH, nursing home; OR, odds ratio; SNF, skilled nursing facility.

was defined as use of more than 5 drugs. In the logistic regression analysis adjusting for demographic, clinical, and staff variables, polypharmacy was associated with increased hospitalization. Patients who were hospitalized were on an average of 6 medications, compared with 3 medications among those who were not hospitalized. Hui and colleageus[56] looked at 606 nursing home patients in Hong Kong. Using multiple logistic regression, they found that polypharmacy ($\geq$5 drugs) was associated with a significantly higher risk of hospitalization over 18 months of follow-up (relative risk, 1.87; 95% CI, 1.06–3.31). Ouslander and colleagues[57] compared Georgia nursing homes with a low hospitalization rate to those with a high hospitalization rate. There was no difference in the percentage of patients on 9 or more medications between these 2 groups of nursing homes. Cooper[58] used the Naranjo algorithm[37] to determine ADRs, and found that patients that had a probable ADR hospitalization were on more medications than those with no ADRs.

Studies of polypharmacy and mortality have demonstrated mixed results. Dedhiya and associates[50] found that polypharmacy was associated with lower mortality, where patients receiving 10 or fewer medications were more likely to die than those receiving more than 10 medications.[50] The authors hypothesized that patients on 10 or fewer medications may have been moribund and possibly in hospice care. Intrator and colleagues[53] reviewed 2080 patients in 1993 using MDS data. Polypharmacy (defined as using >6 medications per week) was not associated with mortality. Leung and co-workers[59] also found no significant association between number of medications and mortality.

Costs of Polypharmacy

The costs of medications among nursing home residents are substantial. A 1999 study of Louisiana nursing home residents determined that the average cost of medications per patient per day was $182, with an estimated annual cost per patient of $2184.[60] However, the average annual drug cost for Veteran long-stay nursing home residents in 2005 was $3629 per resident per year.[61] A 2004 study of nursing home Medicaid beneficiaries in North Carolina found even higher medication costs of $502.96 per month, or approximately $6000 per year.[62,63] A study of drug utilization in Belgian nursing homes found that mean expenditure for chronic medication was 140 EUR per patient per month.[64]

The cost of pharmaceutical services for elderly Medicaid beneficiaries living in nursing homes positively correlated with the number of inappropriate drugs prescribed.[65] However, this study was conducted in 1996 and the costs of drugs have since increased.

Additional factors are important to consider when examining costs of medications. In 1997, experts estimated that for every $1 spent on drugs in nursing facilities, $1.33 was spent on drug-related morbidity and mortality, resulting in $3 billion in drug costs, and an additional $4 billion in estimated healthcare costs of drug-related morbidity and mortality.[66] A 2001 update of drug costs in ambulatory care reflected that costs had more than doubled since 1995,[67] but no updates have been published for nursing home patient drug costs.

Another important factor to consider is the cost to the facility for staff time for medication passes. Nursing and nurse aide expenses are a significant component of nursing home costs.[68] Nursing time for medication administration was estimated at 45 seconds for each oral medication pass.[69] The cost of adding an oral medication once a day for a patient was between $7 and $10 depending on timing of administration, and the cost of adding an oral crushed medication once a day was between $21 and $31, depending on whether the medication was given at an existing medication pass or a new medication pass needed to be added.[69]

Nursing medication administration times also differed, depending on type of nursing home unit (62 minutes per 20 residents on physical support units, vs 84 minutes per 20 residents on behavioral care units). Times also differed depending on whether the nurse was a regular (68 minutes per 20 residents) versus temporary employee (90 minutes per 20 residents).[70] An intervention to eliminate an evening mealtime medication pass at a nursing home decreased the total amount of time spent passing medications from 29.8 to 21.3 minutes per resident per day, representing an average savings of 28% in nursing time per day.[71]

The cost of drug wastage also adds to the overall cost of medication use in nursing home facilities. To the authors' knowledge, there are no recent studies on this subject in nursing homes.

Role of Pharmacists

Consultant pharmacists have been used in nursing homes to enhance patient safety and manage medication costs. Consultant pharmacists began quarterly drug regimen reviews in 1974. After the Omnibus Budget Reconciliation Act of 1987, monthly drug regimen reviews became mandatory.[63,72,73] In July 1999, the Centers for Medicare and Medicaid Services mandated expansions to the drug use review policy for nursing home certification.[74] These monthly drug regimen reviews were determined to be effective.

In 1995, the Fleetwood Model was proposed as an alternative mode for nursing home clinical pharmacy services. This model involved prospective instead of retrospective drug regimen reviews, required direct communication with prescribers, and formalized medication planning for patients at highest risk for medication-related problems. It has been shown to save $3.6 billion annually in costs from avoidance of medication-related problems,[66] is feasible,[75] and resulted in creation of computer software for medication care planning,[76] treatment algorithms with alternative treatments, and ways to eliminate duplicate steps in medication administration. The Fleetwood Model of pharmacists interacting with the interdisciplinary care team has resulted in a more efficient process within nursing facility pharmacies, with more clinical involvement of pharmacists, improved communication with the interdisciplinary team and more time spent on pharmaceutical care planning.[77]

Studies on outcomes of the role of the consultant pharmacist in the nursing home have been mixed. One study cited unclear effectiveness of drug regimen reviews to improve patient safety in nursing homes.[74] A recent review of pharmacist interventions in nursing homes outside the United States had mixed results. They concluded that the acceptance of the pharmacists' recommendations by physicians seems to be essential to have an effect, and that more research is needed in this area.[72] One study estimated that the cost of drug-related morbidity and mortality with the services of consultant pharmacists was $4 billion, compared with $7.6 billion without the services of consultant pharmacists.[66] A systematic review found that interventions led by pharmacists were effective, but the actual reduction in the number of medications was small.[78] Medication change rates owing to consultant pharmacist recommendation ranged from 46% to 68%, and change rate was 73% when physicians, care managers and participants/caregivers were all contacted by pharmacists.[79] One study in 204 geriatric nursing home patients found that acceptance of consultant pharmacist drug therapy recommendations from monthly drug regimen reviews saved $223,218, whereas potential cost savings from recommendations that were rejected were $224,593 over 2 years.[80]

For nursing home certification, state surveyors and consultant pharmacists examine the facility records for potentially inappropriate medication use and medication-related adverse reactions. Noncompliance may result in citations for deficient care.[74] Changes in the Pharmacy Services Tags (F425, F428, F431) and Unnecessary Medications Tag (F329) in the interpretive guidelines released by the Centers for Medicare and Medicaid Services impact the work of consultant pharmacists.[77]

There have been multiple studies of successful interventions to reduce polypharmacy in nursing homes, and to reduce the cost of medications in nursing home residents. A drug therapy management service reduced polypharmacy in North Carolina Medicaid recipients who were high users of prescription drugs, and saved a mean of $30.33 per patient per month initially.[63] Among the non–high-risk, overall nursing home patient population, the intervention saved $21.63 per Medicaid member per month in drug costs.[81] The cost savings varied by whether the pharmacist provided a recommendation, and whether or not the recommendation was accepted. The patients with change in therapy as a result of acceptance of pharmacist recommendation had a mean savings of $20.56 per patient per month, whereas the comparison group patients' medication costs increased by $15 per patient per month during the intervention period.[62]

A randomized, controlled trial of a clinical pharmacy intervention in Australian nursing homes reduced drug use with no change in morbidity or mortality. Estimates of annual medication cost savings owing to the intervention were 64 Australian dollars per resident (25 pounds sterling).[82] A case conference intervention involving a multidisciplinary team of health professionals improved medication appropriateness among residents with medication problems, challenging behaviors, or both.[83] A randomized, controlled trial of pharmacist medication reviews in nursing homes reduced the number of drugs prescribed, with a smaller number of deaths in the intervention period.[84]

A pharmacist intervention for nursing home residents receiving nonsteroidal anti-inflammatory drug or acetaminophen therapy for osteoarthritis provided recommendations to treating physicians regarding monitoring and substitution of nonsteroidal anti-inflammatory drugs with acetaminophen. Eleven patients' physicians rejected the pharmacist recommendations; of these, 5 developed gastrointestinal bleeding requiring 6 hospitalizations and resulting in 2 deaths. The study estimated cost savings for acetaminophen substitution in the intervention rejection group would exceed $91,000, whereas the cost savings with the addition of monitoring for anemia would exceed $84,200.[85]

Some studies have demonstrated limited effectiveness of interventions to reduce medication costs in nursing homes. Multidisciplinary case conference reviews in 3 Australian nursing homes resulted in nonsignificant reductions in medication orders, costs, and mortality, but the physicians and directors of nursing had positive responses to the reviews.[86] The addition of a pharmacist transition coordinator for older adults moving from hospital to nursing home facility reduced worsening pain, but had no effect on hospital readmissions or ADEs.[87]

The costs of hospitalizations related to polypharmacy and inappropriate medication use in nursing home residents is an important area that merits further research. Few studies have examined the costs of hospitalizations due to ADRs, and these studies were not limited to nursing home patients. A 2003 US study of drug-related emergency department visits for elderly veterans found that the total cost of drug-related emergency department visits and hospitalizations was approximately $1.5 million over 12 weeks.[88] In an English study, the projected annual cost of hospital admissions for ADRs was $847 million dollars per year.[89] A 2001 meta-analysis estimated that the costs of preventable ADR-related hospital admissions range between $158 million and $365 million per year.[90] None of these studies examined nursing home residents exclusively. More studies of nursing home patients are needed to better understand the costs of hospitalizations related to medications in this population.

The influence of medical insurance on polypharmacy has had little study. One study of the effect of Medicare Part D on prescribing patterns found that beneficiaries received 7% to 30% fewer medication administrations during skilled nursing facility months (without part D coverage, only Part A) compared with months spent only in other long-term care facility stays (with Part D coverage).[91]

SUMMARY

This article provides a comprehensive review of the outcomes of polypharmacy in nursing homes. Our review had some limitations. First, we only included studies beginning in 1990, and significant earlier studies are not included. Only English-language articles were included. We only researched studies from MEDLINE, and may have missed studies based on our search terms and search tools. There are many definitions of polypharmacy in the literature, including number of medications or inappropriate medications. In this review, we defined polypharmacy as a high number of medications, but not inappropriate medications.

It was not surprising that polypharmacy was consistently associated with an increased number of potentially inappropriate drugs. The majority of studies we reviewed showed that polypharmacy was associated with increased ADEs, increased DDIs, and increased hospitalizations. We were surprised that polypharmacy was not consistently linked with falls, fractures, and mortality. For the mortality studies, it has been postulated that perhaps some patients receiving 10 or more medications may have been moribund or receiving end-of-life or hospice care. It is possible that the number of medications is not as important as the number of potentially inappropriate drugs. There need to be more studies on these outcomes, using different definitions of polypharmacy.

Polypharmacy was associated with increased costs. The drug-related morbidity and mortality, including those resulting from inappropriate medications and increased staff time, led to increased costs. Use of consultant pharmacists has been shown to decrease polypharmacy costs.

DISCLOSURES

This research was supported by The John A. Hartford Foundation Center of Excellence in Geriatrics, University of Hawaii; the funding sources had no role in the analysis and preparation of this paper. Dr Bell received compensation for participation in Aloha Care, a local insurance company Pharmacy and Therapeutics committee. Drs Tamura, Inaba and Masaki have no conflicts to declare.

REFERENCES

1. Lau DT, Kasper JD, Potter DE, et al. Potentially inappropriate medication prescriptions among elderly nursing home residents: their scope and associated resident and facility characteristics. Health Serv Res 2004;39:1257–76.
2. Tamura BK, Bell CL, Lubimir K, et al. Physician intervention for medication reduction in a nursing home: the polypharmacy outcomes project. J Am Med Dir Assoc 2011;12:326–30.

3. O'Mahony D, Gallagher PF. Inappropriate prescribing in the older population: need for new criteria. Age Ageing 2008;37:138–41.

4. Gallagher P, Barry P, O'Mahony D. Inappropriate prescribing in the elderly. J Clin Pharm Ther 2007;32:113–21.

5. Hanlon JT, Shimp LA, Semla TP. Recent advances in geriatrics: drug-related problems in the elderly. Ann Pharmacother 2000;34:360–5.

6. Ruggiero C, Dell'Aquila G, Gasperini B, et al. Potentially inappropriate drug prescriptions and risk of hospitalization among older, Italian, nursing home residents: the ULISSE project. Drugs Aging 2010;27:747–58.

7. Dhall J, Larrat EP, Lapane KL. Use of potentially inappropriate drugs in nursing homes. Pharmacotherapy 2002;22:88–96.

8. Beers MH. Explicit criteria for determining potentially inappropriate medication use by the elderly. An update. Arch Intern Med 1997;157:1531–6.

9. Williams B, Betley C. Inappropriate use of nonpsychotropic medications in nursing homes. J Am Geriatr Soc 1995;43:513–9.

10. Beers MH, Ouslander JG, Rollingher I, et al. Explicit criteria for determining inappropriate medication use in nursing home residents. UCLA Division of Geriatric Medicine. Arch Intern Med 1991;151:1825–32.

11. Rancourt C, Moisan J, Baillargeon L, et al. Potentially inappropriate prescriptions for older patients in long-term care. BMC Geriatr 2004;4:9.

12. Beers MH, Ouslander JG, Fingold SF, et al. Inappropriate medication prescribing in skilled-nursing facilities. Ann Intern Med 1992;117:684–9.

13. McLeod PJ, Huang AR, Tamblyn RM, et al. Defining inappropriate practices in prescribing for elderly people: a national consensus panel. CMAJ 1997;156:385–91.

14. Stafford AC, Alswayan MS, Tenni PC. Inappropriate prescribing in older residents of Australian care homes. J Clin Pharm Ther 2011;36:33–44.

15. Fick DM, Cooper JW, Wade WE, et al. Updating the Beers criteria for potentially inappropriate medication use in older adults: results of a US consensus panel of experts. Arch Intern Med 2003;163:2716–24.

16. Hosia-Randell HM, Muurinen SM, Pitkala KH. Exposure to potentially inappropriate drugs and drug–drug interactions in elderly nursing home residents in Helsinki, Finland: a cross-sectional study. Drugs Aging 2008;25:683–92.

17. Niwata S, Yamada Y, Ikegami N. Prevalence of inappropriate medication using Beers criteria in Japanese long-term care facilities. BMC Geriatr 2006;6:1.

18. Perri M 3rd, Menon AM, Deshpande AD, et al. Adverse outcomes associated with inappropriate drug use in nursing homes. Ann Pharmacother 2005;39:405–11.

19. Nygaard HA, Naik M, Ruths S, et al. Nursing-home residents and their drug use: a comparison between mentally intact and mentally impaired residents. The Bergen district nursing home (BEDNURS) study. Eur J Clin Pharmacol 2003;59:463–9.

20. Mamun K, Lien CT, Goh-Tan CY, et al. Polypharmacy and inappropriate medication use in Singapore nursing homes. Ann Acad Med Singapore 2004;33:49–52.

21. Strand LM, Morley PC, Cipolle RJ, et al. Drug-related problems: their structure and function. DICP 1990;24:1093–7.

22. Chiang L, Hirsch SH, Reuben DB. Predictors of medication prescription in nursing homes. J Am Med Dir Assoc 2000;1:97–102.

23. Gill SS, Misiaszek BC, Brymer C. Improving prescribing in the elderly: a study in the long term care setting. Can J Clin Pharmacol 2001;8:78–83.

24. Naugler CT, Brymer C, Stolee P, et al. Development and validation of an improving prescribing in the elderly tool. Can J Clin Pharmacol 2000;7:103–7.

25. Charlson ME, Pompei P, Ales KL, et al. A new method of classifying prognostic comorbidity in longitudinal studies: development and validation. J Chronic Dis 1987; 40:373–83.
26. Snowdon J, Day S, Baker W. Audits of medication use in Sydney nursing homes. Age Ageing 2006;35:403–8.
27. Balogun S. PM, Evans J. Potentially inappropriate medications in nursing homes: sources and correlates. Internet Journal of Geriatrics and Gerontology 2005;2.
28. Hanlon JT, Schmader KE, Ruby CM, et al. Suboptimal prescribing in older inpatients and outpatients. J Am Geriatr Soc 2001;49:200–9.
29. Hanlon JT, Schmader KE, Koronkowski MJ, et al. Adverse drug events in high risk older outpatients. J Am Geriatr Soc 1997;45:945–8.
30. Jha AK, Kuperman GJ, Teich JM, et al. Identifying adverse drug events: development of a computer-based monitor and comparison with chart review and stimulated voluntary report. J Am Med Inform Assoc 1998;5:305–14.
31. Nguyen JK, Fouts MM, Kotabe SE, et al. Polypharmacy as a risk factor for adverse drug reactions in geriatric nursing home residents. Am J Geriatr Pharmacother 2006;4:36–41.
32. Field TS, Gurwitz JH, Avorn J, et al. Risk factors for adverse drug events among nursing home residents. Arch Intern Med 2001;161:1629–34.
33. Gurwitz JH, Sanchez-Cross MT, Eckler MA, et al. The epidemiology of adverse and unexpected events in the long-term care setting. J Am Geriatr Soc 1994;42:33–8.
34. Ruths S, Straand J, Nygaard HA. Multidisciplinary medication review in nursing home residents: what are the most significant drug-related problems? The Bergen District Nursing Home (BEDNURS) study. Qual Saf Health Care 2003;12:176–80.
35. Busto U, Naranjo CA, Sellers EM. Comparison of two recently published algorithms for assessing the probability of adverse drug reactions. Br J Clin Pharmacol 1982;13: 223–7.
36. Lanctot KL, Naranjo CA. Comparison of the Bayesian approach and a simple algorithm for assessment of adverse drug events. Clin Pharmacol Ther 1995;58: 692–8.
37. Naranjo CA, Busto U, Sellers EM, et al. A method for estimating the probability of adverse drug reactions. Clin Pharmacol Ther 1981;30:239–45.
38. Cooper JW. Probable adverse drug reactions in a rural geriatric nursing home population: a four-year study. J Am Geriatr Soc 1996;44:194–7.
39. Gerety MB, Cornell JE, Plichta DT, et al. Adverse events related to drugs and drug withdrawal in nursing home residents. J Am Geriatr Soc 1993;41:1326–32.
40. Liao HL, Chen JT, Ma TC, et al. Analysis of drug–drug interactions (DDIs) in nursing homes in Central Taiwan. Arch Gerontol Geriatr 2008;47:99–107.
41. Kannus P, Parkkari J, Niemi S, et al. Fall-induced deaths among elderly people. Am J Public Health 2005;95:422–4.
42. Vu MQ, Weintraub N, Rubenstein LZ. Falls in the nursing home: Are they preventable? J Am Med Dir Assoc 2005;6(3 Suppl):S82–7.
43. Baranzini F, Diurni M, Ceccon F, et al. Fall-related injuries in a nursing home setting: is polypharmacy a risk factor? BMC Health Serv Res 2009;9:228.
44. Ruthazer R, Lipsitz LA. Antidepressants and falls among elderly people in long-term care. Am J Public Health 1993;83:746–9.
45. Yip YB, Cumming RG. The association between medications and falls in Australian nursing-home residents. Med J Aust 1994;160:14–8.
46. Lipsitz LA, Jonsson PV, Kelley MM, et al. Causes and correlates of recurrent falls in ambulatory frail elderly. J Gerontol 1991;46:M114–22.

47. Kerman M, Mulvihill M. The role of medication in falls among the elderly in a long-term care facility. Mt Sinai J Med 1990;57:343–7.

48. Chen JS, Sambrook PN, Simpson JM, et al. Risk factors for hip fracture among institutionalised older people. Age Ageing 2009;38:429–34.

49. Chen JS, Simpson JM, March LM, et al. Fracture risk assessment in frail older people using clinical risk factors. Age Ageing 2008;37:536–41.

50. Dedhiya SD, Hancock E, Craig BA, et al. Incident use and outcomes associated with potentially inappropriate medication use in older adults. Am J Geriatr Pharmacother 2010;8:562–70.

51. Mathew R, Young Y, Shrestha S. Factors associated with potentially preventable hospitalization among nursing home residents in New York state with chronic kidney disease. J Am Med Dir Assoc 2011. [Epub ahead of print].

52. Grabowski DC, O'Malley AJ, Barhydt NR. The costs and potential savings associated with nursing home hospitalizations. Health Affairs 2007;26:1753–61.

53. Intrator O, Castle NG, Mor V. Facility characteristics associated with hospitalization of nursing home residents: results of a national study. Med Care 1999;37:228–37.

54. Tang M, Woo J, Hui E, et al. Utilization of emergency room and hospitalization by Chinese nursing home residents: a cross-sectional study. J Am Med Dir Assoc 2010;11:325–32.

55. Cherubini A, Eusebi P, Dell'aquila G, et al. Predictors of Hospitalization in Italian Nursing Home Residents: The U.L.I.S.S.E. Project. J Am Med Dir Assoc 2011. [Epub ahead of print].

56. Hui E, Wong E, Woo, J. Predictors of hospitalization and death in nursing home residents. Hong Kong Journal of Gerontology 2000;14:63–5.

57. Ouslander JG, Lamb G, Perloe M, et al. Potentially avoidable hospitalizations of nursing home residents: frequency, causes, and costs [see editorial comments by Drs. Jean F. Wyman and William R. Hazzard, pp 760–1]. J Am Geriatr Soc 2010;58:627–35.

58. Cooper JW. Adverse drug reaction-related hospitalizations of nursing facility patients: a 4-year study. South Med J 1999;92:485–90.

59. Leung KK, Tang LY, Lue BH. Self-rated health and mortality in Chinese institutional elderly persons. J Clin Epidemiol 1997;50:1107–16.

60. Kamboj S, Kumar P, Cai X, et al. Cost of medications for elderly in a nursing home. Journal of the Louisiana State Medical Society 1999;151:470–2.

61. French DD, Campbell RR, Spehar AM, et al. Drug costs and use in VHA nursing homes: a national overview of long-stay residents. J Am Med Dir Assoc 2007;8:515–8.

62. Trygstad TK, Christensen D, Garmise J, et al. Pharmacist response to alerts generated from Medicaid pharmacy claims in a long-term care setting: results from the North Carolina polypharmacy initiative. J Manag Care Pharm 2005;11:575–83.

63. Christensen D, Trygstad T, Sullivan R, et al. A pharmacy management intervention for optimizing drug therapy for nursing home patients. Am J Geriatr Pharmacother 2004;2:248–56.

64. Elseviers MM, Vander Stichele RR, Van Bortel L. Drug utilization in Belgian nursing homes: impact of residents' and institutional characteristics. Pharmacoepidemiol Drug Saf 2010;19:1041–8.

65. Gupta S, Rappaport HM, Bennett LT. Inappropriate drug prescribing and related outcomes for elderly Medicaid beneficiaries residing in nursing homes. Clin Ther 1996;18:183–96.

66. Bootman JL, Harrison DL, Cox E. The health care cost of drug-related morbidity and mortality in nursing facilities. Arch Intern Med 1997;157:2089–96.

67. Ernst FR, Grizzle AJ. Drug-related morbidity and mortality: updating the cost-of-illness model. J Am Pharm Assoc (Wash) 2001;41:192–9.
68. Hicks LL, Rantz MJ, Petroski GF, et al. Assessing contributors to cost of care in nursing homes. Nursing Economics 1997;15:205–12.
69. Hamrick I, Nye AM, Gardner CK. Nursing home medication administration cost minimization analysis. J Am Med Dir Assoc 2007;8:173–7.
70. Thomson MS, Gruneir A, Lee M, et al. Nursing time devoted to medication administration in long-term care: clinical, safety, and resource implications. J Am Geriatr Soc 2009;57:266–72.
71. Liebel DV, Watson N. Consolidating medication passes: it can lead to more time with patients. Am J Nurs 2005;105:63–4.
72. Verrue CL, Petrovic M, Mehuys E, et al. Pharmacists' interventions for optimization of medication use in nursing homes: a systematic review. Drugs Aging 2009;26:37–49.
73. Levenson SA, Saffel D. The consultant pharmacist and the physician in the nursing home: roles, relationships, and a recipe for success. Consult Pharm 2007;22:71–82.
74. Briesacher B, Limcangco R, Simoni-Wastila L, et al. Evaluation of nationally mandated drug use reviews to improve patient safety in nursing homes: a natural experiment. J Am Geriatr Soc 2005;53:991–6.
75. Lapane KL, Hughes CM. Pharmacotherapy interventions undertaken by pharmacists in the Fleetwood phase III study: the role of process control. Ann Pharmacother 2006;40:1522–6.
76. Lapane KL, Hiris J, Hughes CM, et al. Development and implementation of pharmaceutical care planning software for nursing homes based on the Fleetwood Model. Am J Health Syst Pharm 2006;63:2483–7.
77. Bain KT. Adverse drug reactions and current state of drug regimen review in nursing facilities: need for a change? Consult Pharm 2007;22:586–92.
78. Rollason V, Vogt N. Reduction of polypharmacy in the elderly: a systematic review of the role of the pharmacist. Drugs Aging 2003;20:817–32.
79. Alkema GE, Enguidanos SM, Wilber KH, et al. The role of consultant pharmacists in reducing medication problems among older adults receiving Medicaid waiver services. Consult Pharm 2009;24:121–33.
80. Cooper JW Jr. Consultant pharmacist drug therapy recommendations from monthly drug regimen reviews in a geriatric nursing facility: a two-year study and cost analysis. J Nutr Health Aging 1997;1:181–4.
81. Trygstad TK, Christensen DB, Wegner SE, et al. Analysis of the North Carolina long-term care polypharmacy initiative: a multiple-cohort approach using propensity-score matching for both evaluation and targeting. Clin Ther 2009;31:2018–37.
82. Roberts MS, Stokes JA, King MA, et al. Outcomes of a randomized controlled trial of a clinical pharmacy intervention in 52 nursing homes. Br J Clin Pharmacol 2001;51:257–65.
83. Crotty M, Halbert J, Rowett D, et al. An outreach geriatric medication advisory service in residential aged care: a randomised controlled trial of case conferencing. Age Ageing 2004;33:612–7.
84. Furniss L, Burns A, Craig SK, et al. Effects of a pharmacist's medication review in nursing homes. Randomised controlled trial. Br J Psychiatry 2000;176:563–7.
85. Cooper JW, Wade WE. Pharmacist interventions in geriatric nursing facility NSAID therapy: a one-year follow-up study of costs and outcomes. Consult Pharm 2005;20:492–7.
86. King MA, Roberts MS. Multidisciplinary case conference reviews: improving outcomes for nursing home residents, carers and health professionals. Pharm World Sci 2001;23:41–5.

87. Crotty M, Rowett D, Spurling L, et al. Does the addition of a pharmacist transition coordinator improve evidence-based medication management and health outcomes in older adults moving from the hospital to a long-term care facility? Results of a randomized, controlled trial. Am J Geriatr Pharmacother 2004;2:257–64.

88. Yee JL, Hasson NK, Schreiber DH. Drug-related emergency department visits in an elderly veteran population. Ann Pharmacother 2005;39:1990–5.

89. Pirmohamed M, Darbyshire J. Collecting and sharing information about harms. BMJ 2004;329:6–7.

90. Beijer HJ, de Blaey CJ. Hospitalisations caused by adverse drug reactions (ADR): a meta-analysis of observational studies. Pharm World Sci 2002;24:46–54.

91. Stuart B, Simoni-Wastila L, Shaffer T. Medication patterns for Medicare beneficiaries with SNF/LTC facility stays. Health Care Financing Review 2008;29:13–25.

Deprescribing Trials: Methods to Reduce Polypharmacy and the Impact on Prescribing and Clinical Outcomes

Danijela Gnjidic, PhD, MPH[a,b,c,*], David G. Le Couteur, MBBS, PhD[b,c,d], Lisa Kouladjian, BMedSc (Hons), MPharm[a], Sarah N. Hilmer, MBBS, PhD[a,b]

KEYWORDS

- Effectiveness of interventions • Medications • Polypharmacy
- Medication withdrawal • Older adults

THE RISKS OF POLYPHARMACY

There are many challenges to ensuring good outcomes from the pharmacologic management of older adults. With advancing age, the increased prevalence of diseases promotes high use of medications in older adults and of polypharmacy, commonly defined as the use of 5 or more medications. Further, there is a lack of data to guide the use of medications in older adults. This is because older adults are rarely included in randomized, controlled trials (RCT),[1] and most evidence-based clinical guidelines for older people are extrapolated from younger populations.[2] Older adults use medicines extensively, and evidence suggests that polypharmacy may even be increasing.[3] For instance, older people living in the community consume on average 4 medications, whereas older people living in nursing homes use on average 7 medications.[4–6]

Many risk factors for polypharmacy have been identified, commonly grouped as demographic, health status, and access to health care services factors.[7] Of demographic

---

Disclosures: The authors gratefully acknowledge the funding support from the Geoff and Elaine Penney Ageing Research Unit and the Ageing and Alzheimer's Research Foundation.

[a] Departments of Clinical Pharmacology and Aged Care, 11C Main Building, Royal North Shore Hospital, St Leonards NSW 2065, Australia
[b] Sydney Medical School, University of Sydney, Sydney, NSW 2006, Australia
[c] Centre for Education and Research on Ageing, Concord Hospital, C22, Concord NSW 2139, Australia
[d] ANZAC Medical Research Institute, Concord Hospital and University of Sydney, Concord NSW 2139, Australia
* Corresponding author. Sydney Medical School, University of Sydney, Sydney, NSW 2006, Australia.
E-mail address: danijela.gnjidic@sydney.edu.au

risk factors, advancing age, female gender, and low education level are associated with increased polypharmacy exposure.[3,7–9] Recent hospitalization, multiple comorbidities, and depression are some of the health status markers associated with higher rates of polypharmacy.[9] The involvement of multiple prescribers and greater health care utilization are important health care characteristics that increase the risk of polypharmacy.[8] A recent study conducted in a sample of older disabled women found that in addition to comorbidity and difficulties with instrumental activities of daily living, frailty was associated with increased polypharmacy.[10]

Although use of multiple medications might generate positive outcomes for some older adults with multiple diseases, there is increasing evidence that it is associated with increased risks of adverse events. The clinical consequences of polypharmacy on health outcomes in older adults have been widely documented. Polypharmacy is associated with increased risks of adverse drug reactions (ADRs), adverse drug events (ADEs), inappropriate prescribing, inappropriate drug use, falls, hospitalization, institutionalization, mortality, and other important negative outcomes in studies of older adults.[6,11] Indeed, polypharmacy is often considered to be among the most important risk factors for ADRs in older people. Therefore, rational withdrawal of medications may be the appropriate clinical decision and may result in significant clinical and functional benefits in some older people with polypharmacy. The feasibility of deprescribing was recently evaluated in a pilot study,[12] where it was found that a RCT of deprescribing is acceptable to participants, and recruitment is feasible. Current evidence suggests that stopping some classes of medications in older patients does not worsen clinical outcomes, is not often associated with withdrawal syndromes, and can improve some outcomes such as falls, behavior, and cognition.[13]

Not surprisingly, withdrawing medications in older people has often been found to be difficult, and requires consideration of a range of factors. To date, interventions to reduce medication exposure in older adults have shown mixed results. Approaches including pharmacist-led medication reviews, prescriber feedback, and multidisciplinary interventions involving a team of health professionals have been trialed to reduce medications, with the aim of improving medication-related outcomes in older adults. The clinical implications of different interventions in older people from care homes,[14] and pharmacist-based interventions to optimize prescribing in older adults,[15] especially for those living in nursing homes[16,17] have been evaluated recently. The aim of this clinical review is to highlight the evidence for the impact of various types of interventions designed to reduce polypharmacy on prescribing and clinical outcomes in older adults from community, nursing home, and hospital settings.

CHALLENGES OF DISCONTINUING MEDICATIONS

Before addressing interventions to reduce medications in older adults, it is important to briefly discuss factors that need to be considered during the medication withdrawal process (Fig. 1). There are many barriers to successfully stopping medications in older adults. Health professionals may find it difficult to reduce the dose or to stop the medication once a prescription is initiated. Clinicians might feel uncomfortable with changing or discontinuing a medication prescribed by another clinician.[18] The evidence base, marketing, and guidelines for initiating medications are vast, but there is little to support ceasing or reducing medications. Patients' preferences are also important to consider before initiating the process of medication withdrawal. Patients may be psychologically and physically attached to their medications.[19] Stopping a medication may be perceived by the patient or their carer/family as inadequate care. The relationship between the health professionals and patient may hinder the efforts to stop medicines.

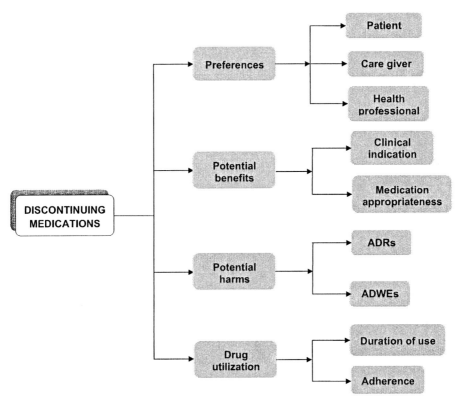

Fig. 1. Factors to consider when discontinuing medications in older adults. ADRs, adverse drug interactions; ADWEs, adverse drug withdrawal events.

The potential harms of discontinuing medications may be a barrier to successful medication withdrawal process. The process of stopping medications can result in ADRs or adverse drug withdrawal events (ADWEs). An ADWE is characterized by a clinically significant set of symptoms or signs caused by the medication cessation.[20] Some medications are more likely to cause ADWEs than others. For example, the cardiovascular and central nervous system drug classes are the most common medications associated with ADWEs.[20,21]

When considering whether to continue or withdraw a patient's medicines, it is important to establish duration of use of each medication, whether there is still an indication for the use of medication, and if so, the use is still consistent with current guidelines.[22] Medication adherence is another important factor that might impact on attempts to withdraw medications.[23] For example, if the patient has remained well without taking the medicine, then it is pointless to continue prescribing the medications. The so-termed prescribing cascade, when additional medicines are initiated to treat adverse effects of other medications, might influence attempts to cease medications, as the adverse effects of remaining drugs will reemerge.[24]

There is very limited evidence to guide the medication withdrawal process in older adults with polypharmacy. An algorithm approach that expands the prescribing stage to include a step for rationally discontinuing medications has been proposed.[19] In clinical practice, a step-wise approach to discontinuing medications is

Table 1
Clinical controlled studies to reduce medication exposure

Intervention	Study Setting[a]	Study Results	
		Impact on Prescribing	Impact on Outcomes
Pharmacist-based interventions			
Clinical pharmacist medication review combined with physician and patient education[26]	Outpatient managed care (n = 195,971)	Significant reduction in the number of prescriptions	Not assessed
Clinical pharmacist consultation and computer-based medication profiles provided to physician[27]	Internal medicine clinic (n = 512)	Significant reduction in the number of medications	Not assessed
Clinical pharmacist patient tailored medication review provided to physician[28]	Outpatient clinic (n = 562)	Significant reduction in the number and costs of medications	Not assessed
Medication review performed by pharmacist and reviewed by the primary care provider[29]	Geriatric outpatient clinic (n = 250)	Significant reduction in the mean number of medications	Neutral or positive in 99.5% of cases
Physician-based interventions			
The Good Palliative–Geriatric Practice algorithm compromised of physician individual review[30]	Community dwelling (n = 75)	Discontinued 311 medications (58%) in 64 participants	Improved cognition and global health
Prompting participants to bring their medications for review by their physician[31]	Managed care organization (n = 37,372)	Significant reduction in the number of medications observed in 20% of patients	Not assessed

Geriatric medicine fellows reviewed each patient's medication list, and recommended the changes to the patients' primary care physician[32]	Nursing homes (n = 74)	Significant reduction in the number of medications	Not assessed
Provision of admission medication list to physician[33]	Hospitalized patients (n = 836)	Significant reduction in the number of medications	Not assessed
Multidisciplinary-based interventions			
Clinical pharmacists prescribed medications under the supervision of a family physician[34]	Nursing homes (n = 139)	Pharmacists prescribed significantly less medications than physicians	Improved survival (P = .05); more patients discharged to lower levels of care (P = .03)
Case conference involving health professionals including general practitioner, pharmacist, nurses and other health professional[35]	Nursing home (n = 245)	Nonsignificant reduction in the number of medications	No effect on mortality

[a] N refers to number of patient participants.

usually recommended.[22,25] A gradual tapering of a dose, particularly for medications used on a long-term basis and those associated with withdrawal syndromes is often recommended. If the process of medication withdrawal is undertaken slowly and under appropriate supervision, the likelihood of clinically significant ADWEs is low.[13]

INTERVENTIONS TO REDUCE MEDICATIONS: IMPACT ON PRESCRIBING AND OUTCOMES

A number of clinical controlled studies have been performed to assess the effectiveness of various interventions to reduce medication exposure in older adults (**Table 1**). These approaches have commonly included medication reviews delivered by clinical pharmacists, prescriber education programs, academic detailing combined with additional strategies, comprehensive geriatric assessments, and multidisciplinary interventions engaging health professionals such as physicians and pharmacists.

Of 4 clinical studies that involved pharmacist-based interventions, all reduced polypharmacy, but only one assessed the impact of medication reduction on clinical outcomes. One intervention, compromising of a clinical pharmacist medication review combined with physician and patient education, resulted in significant reductions in number of prescriptions and medication costs.[26] Two identical interventions separated by 1 year were administered in the same study sample. The number of prescriptions decreased from 4.6 to 2.2 after the first intervention and from 4.5 to 4.0 six months after the second intervention. Further, adding a computer-based medication profile during the consultation between clinical pharmacists and physicians results in a significant reduction in the number of medications.[27] The provision of a patient-tailored medication review by pharmacist to physician reduces the number and cost of medications.[28] Medication reviews led by a pharmacist and reviewed by the primary care provider have also been found to result in a significant reduction in the mean number of medications, as well as reduced medication costs.[29] Moreover, the same study reported neutral or positive clinical outcomes of medication-related changes in 99.5% of patients.

Four clinical controlled studies employing physician-based interventions were identified[30–33]; similarly, although all reduced polypharmacy, only 1 study reported the impact of medication reduction on outcomes.[30] A recent trial of polypharmacy reduction in older people showed that over half of medicines can be discontinued.[30] The study utilized the good palliative–geriatric practice algorithm, which involved physician-based reviews. Only 2% of medicines had to be restarted because of recurrence of the original indication and overall there was improvement in cognition and global health. This is a very important study, because it showed that not only can polypharmacy reduction be achieved, but that this is associated with long-term adherence and improved patient outcomes. In a study that promoted medication reviews by primary care physicians with their patients, significant changes in physicians' prescribing practices were observed.[31] Of the 42% of the participants who underwent the medication review by the physician, 20% reported having a medication stopped and 29% reported a change in the dose of a medication. The other 2 studies also demonstrated a significant reduction in the number of medications.[32,33]

Two controlled studies utilizing a multidisciplinary intervention assessed the impact of medication reduction on outcomes. One study compared prescribing practices of the clinical pharmacists, under the supervision of a physician, with the usual care in a nursing home setting.[34] The study found that pharmacists prescribed significantly lower numbers of medications than physicians. Moreover, this was associated with a significantly lower number of deaths ($P = .05$) and a significantly higher number of patients being discharged to lower levels of care ($P = .03$). The other study reported no change in the number of medications or impact on mortality.[35]

DEPRESCRIBING TRIALS TO REDUCE MEDICATIONS: IMPACT ON PRESCRIBING AND OUTCOMES

The studies described in this section represent those which have employed an RCT design to assess the effects of interventions to reduce medicines in older adults. These trials have been conducted in a range of settings, and have yielded mixed results and are summarized in **Table 2**.

RCTs involving medication review performed by pharmacists have been utilized in a few studies.[36–39] Although clinical pharmacist-based interventions have resulted in substantial changes in medication regimens in 2 studies,[36,38] reduced medication use did not seem to cause significant differences in practice consultation rates, outpatient consultations, hospitalization, or mortality. However, a significant reduction in the number of falls over 6 months was reported in 1 study.[38] In a RCT study of pharmacist medication reviews conducted across 14 nursing homes in the UK, reduction in the number of medicines and costs was observed, but was not significant.[39] Further, the number of accidents, falls, or deaths was not different between the groups.

Studies employing physician-based interventions have mostly reported a significant reduction in medication use; however, the impact on clinical outcomes is unclear.[40–43] In 1 study, provision of a comprehensive medication review with recommended modifications of patient's medication regimen to physicians' resulted in a significant reduction in the number of medications and costs, but it did not improve functional outcomes.[40] In 2 studies, the primary outcome was reduction in medication use.[41,42] The application of inpatient or outpatient geriatric evaluation and management seems to be successful in reducing primarily inappropriate drug use and, consequently, the number of medications, with implications in reducing serious ADRs.[43]

A number of studies utilizing multidisciplinary-based interventions across a range of settings have been conducted.[44–54] Two studies implementing multidisciplinary teams of physicians, pharmacists, and nurses reported no difference in the mean number of medications.[44,45] Both studies had a same duration of follow-up and were conducted in older people living in the community. In contrast, a study of hospitalized patients who underwent multidisciplinary expert panel medication review showed that, although the total number of medications per patient per day fell slightly from 11.64 to 11.09 in the intervention group ($P = .04$), there was no difference in mortality or frequency of acute hospital transfers.[52] Two studies involving a team of physicians, pharmacists, and nurses were conducted in older people living in nursing homes.[53,54] Both studies reported a significant decrease in number of medications over 1 year of follow-up[53,54]; however, only 1 assessed the impact on outcomes.[53] Although medication use was reduced by 14.8% in intervention compared with the control group, the study found no change in morbidity or mortality outcomes.[53]

More recently, an electronic medical records-based intervention was trialed to reduce overall medication use, psychoactive medication use, and occurrence of falls in older community-dwelling people.[55] Although the intervention did not result in a reduction in the total number of medications, a significant negative relationship between the intervention and the total number of medications started during the intervention period ($P<.01$), and the total number of psychoactive medications ($P<.05$) was observed. The impact on falls was unclear. Although the use of computerized physician order entry and clinical decision support systems seems to improve medication safety,[56] future research is warranted to assess the feasibility of

Table 2
Randomized clinical trials to reduce medication exposure

			Study Results	
Intervention Type	Study Setting[a]	Duration of Follow-Up	Impact on Prescribing	Impact on Outcomes
Pharmacist-based interventions				
Pharmacist performed medication review, with recommendations made to physician in the case of major changes[36]	Community dwelling (n = 1131)	1 year	The increase in the mean number of repeat medications was significantly lower for intervention (mean difference = 0.2) compared with control group (mean difference = 0.4)	No effect on practice consultation rates, outpatient consultations, hospital admissions, or death rate
Clinical pharmacist intervention involving the patient, with recommendations made to physician[37]	General medicine clinic (n = 208)	1 year	Nonsignificant difference in the mean number of medications	No effect on health-related quality of life
Pharmacist performed medication review and consulted with the patient and carer[38]	Nursing homes (n = 661)	6 months	Significant reduction in the number of repeat medications: 3.1 for intervention compared with 2.4 for control group	Reduction in falls; No effect on consultations rates, hospitalizations, deaths, functional status or cognitive performance
Medication review performed by a pharmacist, with recommendations and follow-up[39]	Nursing homes (n = 330)	8 months	Nonsignificant reduction in the number of medications	Minimal effect on morbidity and mortality

Physician-based interventions

Patient-tailored information recommending medication reduction to primary care physician[40]	Community dwelling (n = 140)	2 months	Significant reduction in the number of medications	No differences in functioning
Patient tailored information recommending medication reduction to primary care physician[41]	Outpatient clinic (n = 272)	6 months	Significant reduction in the mean number of medications	Not assessed
Group 1: Patient-tailored letter recommending medication reduction to primary care physician Group 2: A chart review, calculation of patient compliance, and individualized suggestions for medication reduction to primary care physician[42]	Outpatient clinic (n = 292)	6 months	Significant reduction in the number of medications No significant difference between the type of intervention	Not assessed
Inpatient or outpatient geriatric evaluation and management (GEM)[43]	Inpatient and outpatient veterans care (n = 834)	1 year	Significant reduction in unnecessary and inappropriate drug use, and consequent reduction in number of medications was observed in patients receiving GEM	Reduction in serious ADRs

(continued on next page)

Table 2
(continued)

Intervention Type	Study Setting[a]	Duration of Follow-Up	Study Results	
			Impact on Prescribing	Impact on Outcomes
Multidisciplinary-based interventions				
Multidisciplinary team comprising a physician, pharmacist and nurse reviewed the list of medications in a case conference[44]	Community dwelling (n = 266)	1 year	Nonsignificant reduction in the mean number of medications	Not assessed
Evaluation performed by a nurse and physician[45]	Community dwelling (n = 174)	2.5 months 1 year	Nonsignificant reduction in the number of medications	Not assessed
Personal educational visits by clinical pharmacist to primary care physician[46]	Prescription database[b]	9 months	Reduced prescribing of the target medications by 14%	Not assessed
Pharmacist educated the patient/carer about their medicines, and subsequently met with the general practitioner to reinforce changes[47]	Community dwelling (n = 136)	6 months	Decreased number of medications	No difference in hospital admissions, care home admissions, or deaths
Clinical pharmacists visited physicians; second group were given data comparing their individual prescribing costs to those of their colleagues[48]	General medicine clinic[b]	7 months	Significant reduction in physicians' prescribing costs but no decrease in the number of prescriptions	Not assessed
Clinical pharmacist medication review involving the patient, with recommendations made to physician to reduce medications after discharge[49]	Hospitalized patients (n = 706)	3 months 20 months	Significant difference in the mean number of medications observed at 20 months only	No effect on service use

Intervention	Setting	Duration	Medication outcome	Other outcome
Clinical pharmacist medication review involving the patient, with recommendations made to interdisciplinary team (social worker, dietician, physical therapist, geriatric physician and nurse) to reduce medications after admission to a hospital[50]	Hospitalized patients (n = 436)	3 days 3 months	Increase in number of medications in the intervention groups was lower compared with control at 3 days No difference in the number of medications observed at 3 months	Not assessed
Interdisciplinary geriatric evaluation involving the assessment of patient's medical, functional and psychosocial status[51]	Hospitalized patients (n = 123)	2.5 years	No difference in the mean number of medications	Unclear
Medical assessment by a geriatrician and medication review by a multidisciplinary expert panel (geriatricians, specialist registrars in geriatric medicine, hospital pharmacists and senior nurse practitioners)[52]	Hospitalized patients (n = 225)	6 months	Total number of medications reduced in intervention compared with control group	No effect on mortality or frequency of acute hospital transfers
Medication reviews prepared by the pharmacist; educating nurses on common issues in geriatric pharmacotherapy; geriatrician also considered the medication review[53]	Nursing homes (n = 3230)	1 year	Significant reduction in total number of medications when clustering effect was not accounted for	No effect on morbidity or survival

(continued on next page)

Table 2
(continued)

Intervention Type	Study Setting[a]	Duration of Follow-Up	Study Results	
			Impact on Prescribing	Impact on Outcomes
Case conference involving health professionals including physician, pharmacist, nurses and nursing assistant[54]	Nursing homes (n = 1854)	1 year	Significant reduction in the prescribing of antipsychotics, benzodiazepine hypnotics, and antidepressant medications	Not assessed
Computer feedback-based interventions				
A standardized medication review was conducted and recommendations made to the primary physician via the electronic medical record[55]	Community dwelling (n = 620)	1 year	Nonsignificant reduction in the number of medications	Nonsignificant reduction in falls

Abbreviations: ADRs, adverse drug reactions; GEM, geriatric evaluation and management.
[a] N refers to number of patient participants.
[b] Sample size for patient participants not available.

using electronic medical records-based interventions to reduce medication exposure, and the impact on prescribing and outcomes in older adults.

EFFECTIVENESS OF TRIALS TO REDUCE MEDICATION EXPOSURE

Assessing the effectiveness of a range of interventions on prescribing and clinical benefits is challenging because of the range of outcomes measured across studies, as well as differences in the study designs, settings, and types of interventions (**Fig. 2**). While in some studies the main outcome measure was the surrogate outcome of the change in number of medications, other studies selected more clinically relevant outcomes such as hospitalizations, falls, or mortality. Selecting appropriate clinical outcome measures may be the key to significant changes in medication-related outcomes.[57] Associations between medication exposure and clinical outcomes may differ between older people from different settings, with significant differences even observed between studies in different residential aged care facilities.[58] A reduction in number of medications may not be the most appropriate outcome, because this reflects the quantity not the quality of prescribing and does not reflect the need for clinically indicated medications.[6] The lack of effect of interventions may be due to the methods used to collect outcome data and duration of follow-up. For example, recording outcome data from nursing home records may result in misclassification of outcomes, because it may be difficult to establish the causal relationship between medications and these outcomes.[39,53] Two or 3 months of follow-up may not provide evidence on the long-term impact of the interventions.[40,50]

The type of the intervention appears to affect the outcome in some studies. For instance, multidisciplinary interventions,[47,52] personal contact, or academic detailing with the physician[46] seem to demonstrate more significant impact on reducing prescribing than providing educational material alone. However, multidisciplinary interventions may be resource intensive, and it may be difficult to implement such interventions at the population level. To make these interventions more applicable and generalizable between health professionals and across different settings, the risk assessment tools based on the drugs or drug classes known to increase the risk of adverse events could be used to identify medicines to stop in older adults.[18,59] The inclusion of such risk assessment tools may improve the process of identifying those patients most at risk of the adverse effects of polypharmacy.[60]

SUMMARY

Different styles of interventions can reduce medication exposure in older adults. However, the evidence for their clinical effectiveness and sustainability is conflicting and lacking. There are some data to guide clinicians on which medicines are more likely to be inappropriate in older people, which medicines are more likely to cause ADWEs, and which medicines should be tapered slowly rather than stopped. To reduce the likelihood of clinically significant adverse events, clinicians should undertake a step-wise approach to discontinuing medications and do so under appropriate supervision. Further research to determine the most effective ways to discontinue medications, and to provide a better understanding of the clinical benefits of various interventions is required. Large RCTs evaluating multidisciplinary interventions and clinical outcomes of changes in medicines regimen across different settings are required to confirm the findings of the studies performed so far.

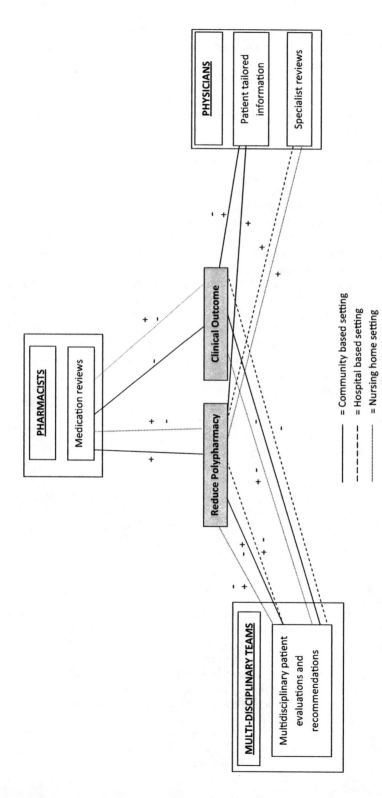

Fig. 2. The impact of methods to reduce medications on polypharmacy exposure and clinical outcomes in older adults. Different line patterns correspond to different study settings. Community based setting includes studies conducted in outpatient clinics. Symbols + (significant reduction in number of medications and/or improved outcomes) or – (non significant effect on number of medications or on outcomes) indicate the impact of methods on polypharmacy and clinical outcomes.

REFERENCES

1. Van Spall HG, Toren A, Kiss A, et al. Eligibility criteria of randomized controlled trials published in high-impact general medical journals: a systematic sampling review. JAMA 2007;297:1233–40.
2. Hilmer SN, Gnjidic D, Abernethy DR. Pharmacoepidemiology in the postmarketing assessment of the efficacy and safety of drugs in older people. J Gerontol A Biol Sci Med Sci 2012;67:181–8.
3. Linjakumpu T, Hartikainen S, Klaukka T, et al. Use of medications and polypharmacy are increasing among the elderly. J Clin Epidemiol 2002;55:809–17.
4. Gnjidic D, Cumming RG, Le Couteur DG, et al. Drug Burden Index and physical function in older Australian men. Br J Clin Pharmacol 2009;68:97–105.
5. Wilson NM, Hilmer SN, March LM, et al. Associations between Drug Burden Index and falls in older people in residential aged care. J Am Geriatr Soc 2011;59:875–80.
6. Hilmer SN, Gnjidic D. The effects of polypharmacy in older adults. Clin Pharmacol Ther 2009;85:86–8.
7. Hajjar ER, Cafiero AC, Hanlon JT. Polypharmacy in elderly patients. Am J Geriatr Pharmacother 2007;5:345–51.
8. Jorgensen T, Johansson S, Kennerfalk A, et al. Prescription drug use, diagnoses, and healthcare utilization among the elderly. Ann Pharmacother 2001;35:1004–9.
9. Bjerrum L, Sogaard J, Hallas J, et al. Polypharmacy: correlations with sex, age and drug regimen. A prescription database study. Eur J Clin Pharmacol 1998;54:197–202.
10. Crentsil V, Ricks MO, Xue QL, et al. A pharmacoepidemiologic study of community-dwelling, disabled older women: factors associated with medication use. J Am Geriatr Soc 2010;8:215–24.
11. Mallet L, Spinewine A, Huang A. The challenge of managing drug interactions in elderly people. Lancet 2007;370:185–91.
12. Beer C, Loh PK, Peng YG, et al. A pilot randomized controlled trial of deprescribing. Ther Adva Drug Saf 2011;2:37–43.
13. Iyer S, Naganathan V, McLachlan AJ, et al. Medication withdrawal trials in people aged 65 years and older: a systematic review. Drugs Aging 2008;25:1021–31.
14. Loganathan M, Singh S, Franklin BD, et al. Interventions to optimise prescribing in care homes: systematic review. Age Ageing 2011;40:150–62.
15. Rollason V, Vogt N. Reduction of polypharmacy in the elderly: a systematic review of the role of the pharmacist. Drugs Aging 2003;20:817–32.
16. Verrue CL, Petrovic M, Mehuys E, et al. Pharmacists' interventions for optimization of medication use in nursing homes: a systematic review. Drugs Aging 2009;26:37–49.
17. Hughes CM, Lapane KL. Pharmacy interventions on prescribing in nursing homes: from evidence to practice. Ther Adva Drug Saf 2011;1–10.
18. Gnjidic D, Le Couteur DG, Abernethy DR, et al. A pilot randomized clinical trial utilizing the drug burden index to reduce exposure to anticholinergic and sedative medications in older people. Ann Pharmacother 2010;44:1725–32.
19. Bain KT, Holmes HM, Beers MH, et al. Discontinuing medications: a novel approach for revising the prescribing stage of the medication-use process. J Am Geriatr Soc 2008;56:1946–52.
20. Graves T, Hanlon JT, Schmader KE, et al. Adverse events after discontinuing medications in elderly outpatients. Arch Intern Med 1997;157:2205–10.
21. Gerety MB, Cornell JE, Plichta DT, et al. Adverse events related to drugs and drug withdrawal in nursing home residents. J Am Geriatr Soc 1993;41:1326–32.

22. Le Couteur DG, Banks E, Gnjidic D, et al. Deprescribing. Australian Prescriber 2011; 34:182–5.

23. MacLaughlin EJ, Raehl CL, Treadway AK, et al. Assessing medication adherence in the elderly: which tools to use in clinical practice? Drugs Aging 2005;22:231–55.

24. Rochon PA, Gurwitz JH. Optimising drug treatment for elderly people: the prescribing cascade. BMJ 1997;315:1096–9.

25. Hardy JE, Hilmer SN. Deprescribing in the last year of life. J Pharm Res 2011;41.

26. Zarowitz BJ, Stebelsky LA, Muma BK, et al. Reduction of high-risk polypharmacy drug combinations in patients in a managed care setting. Pharmacotherapy 2005;25: 1636–45.

27. Tamai IY, Rubenstein LZ, Josephson KR, et al. Impact of computerized drug profiles and a consulting pharmacist on outpatient prescribing patterns: a clinical trial. Drug Intell Clin Pharm 1987;21:890–5.

28. Britton ML, Lurvey PL. Impact of medication profile review on prescribing in a general medicine clinic. Am J Hosp Pharm 1991;48:265–70.

29. Blakey SA, Hixson-Wallace JA. Clinical and economic effects of pharmacy services in geriatric ambulatory clinic. Pharmacotherapy 2000;20:1198–203.

30. Garfinkel D, Mangin D. Feasibility study of a systematic approach for discontinuation of multiple medications in older adults: addressing polypharmacy. Arch Intern Med 2010;170:1648–54.

31. Fillit HM, Futterman R, Orland BI, et al. Polypharmacy management in Medicare managed care: changes in prescribing by primary care physicians resulting from a program promoting medication reviews. Am J Manag Care 1999;5:587–94.

32. Tamura BK, Bell CL, Lubimir K, et al. Physician intervention for medication reduction in a nursing home: the polypharmacy outcomes project. J Am Med Dir Assoc 2011;12:326–30.

33. Muir AJ, Sanders LL, Wilkinson WE, et al. Reducing medication regimen complexity: a controlled trial. J Gen Intern Med 2001;16:77–82.

34. Thompson JF, McGhan WF, Ruffalo RL, et al. Clinical pharmacists prescribing drug therapy in a geriatric setting: outcome of a trial. J Am Geriatr Soc 1984;32:154–9.

35. King MA, Roberts MS. Multidisciplinary case conference reviews: improving outcomes for nursing home residents, carers and health professionals. Pharm World Sci 2001;23:41–5.

36. Zermansky AG, Petty DR, Raynor DK, et al. Randomised controlled trial of clinical medication review by a pharmacist of elderly patients receiving repeat prescriptions in general practice. BMJ 2001;323:1340–3.

37. Hanlon JT, Weinberger M, Samsa GP, et al. A randomized, controlled trial of a clinical pharmacist intervention to improve inappropriate prescribing in elderly outpatients with polypharmacy. Am J Med 1996;100:428–37.

38. Zermansky AG, Alldred DP, Petty DR, et al. Clinical medication review by a pharmacist of elderly people living in care homes-randomised controlled trial. Age Ageing 2006; 35:586–91.

39. Furniss L, Burns A, Craig SK, et al. Effects of a pharmacist's medication review in nursing homes. Randomised controlled trial. Br J Psychiatry 2000;176:563–7.

40. Williams ME, Pulliam CC, Hunter R, et al. The short-term effect of interdisciplinary medication review on function and cost in ambulatory elderly people. J Am Geriatr Soc 2004;52:93–8.

41. Kroenke K, Pinholt EM. Reducing polypharmacy in the elderly. A controlled trial of physician feedback. J Am Geriatr Soc 1990;38:31–6.

42. Meyer TJ, Van Kooten D, Marsh S, et al. Reduction of polypharmacy by feedback to clinicians. J Gen Intern Med 1991;6:133–6.

43. Schmader KE, Hanlon JT, Pieper CF, et al. Effects of geriatric evaluation and management on adverse drug reactions and suboptimal prescribing in the frail elderly. Am J Med 2004;116:394–401.
44. Allard J, Hebert R, Rioux M, et al. Efficacy of a clinical medication review on the number of potentially inappropriate prescriptions prescribed for community-dwelling elderly people. CMAJ 2001;164:1291–6.
45. Pitkala KH, Strandberg TE, Tilvis RS. Is it possible to reduce polypharmacy in the elderly? A randomised, controlled trial. Drugs Aging 2001;18:143–9.
46. Avorn J, Soumerai SB. Improving drug-therapy decisions through educational outreach. A randomized controlled trial of academically based "detailing". N Engl J Med 1983;308:1457–63.
47. Lenaghan E, Holland R, Brooks A. Home-based medication review in a high risk elderly population in primary care-the POLYMED randomised controlled trial. Age Ageing 2007;36:292–7.
48. Steele MA, Bess DT, Franse VL, et al. Cost effectiveness of two interventions for reducing outpatient prescribing costs. DICP 1989;23:497–500.
49. Lipton HL, Bird JA. The impact of clinical pharmacists' consultations on geriatric patients' compliance and medical care use: a randomized controlled trial. Gerontologist 1994;34:307–15.
50. Owens NJ, Sherburne NJ, Silliman RA, et al. The Senior Care Study. The optimal use of medications in acutely ill older patients. J Am Geriatr Soc 1990;38:1082–7.
51. Rubenstein LZ, Josephson K, Wieland GD, et al. Geriatric assessment on a subacute hospital ward. Clin Geriatr Med 1987;3:131–43.
52. Pope G, Wall N, Peters CM, et al. Specialist medication review does not benefit short-term outcomes and net costs in continuing-care patients. Age Ageing 2011;40: 307–12.
53. Roberts MS, Stokes JA, King MA, et al. Outcomes of a randomized controlled trial of a clinical pharmacy intervention in 52 nursing homes. Br J Clin Pharmacol 2001;51: 257–65.
54. Schmidt I, Claesson CB, Westerholm B, et al. The impact of regular multidisciplinary team interventions on psychotropic prescribing in Swedish nursing homes. J Am Geriatr Soc 1998;46:77–82.
55. Weber V, White A, McIlvried R. An electronic medical record (EMR)-based intervention to reduce polypharmacy and falls in an ambulatory rural elderly population. J Gen Intern Med 2008;23:399–404.
56. Kaushal R, Shojania KG, Bates DW. Effects of computerized physician order entry and clinical decision support systems on medication safety: a systematic review. Arch Intern Med 2003;163:1409–16.
57. Majumdar SR, Soumerai SB. Why most interventions to improve physician prescribing do not seem to work. CMAJ 2003;169:30–1.
58. Wilson N, Gnjidic D, March L, et al. Use of PPIs are not associated with mortality in institutionalized older people. Arch Intern Med 2011;171:866.
59. Gallagher PF, O'Connor MN, O'Mahony D. Prevention of potentially inappropriate prescribing for elderly patients: a randomized controlled trial using STOPP/START criteria. Clin Pharmacol Ther 2011;89:845–54.
60. Gnjidic D, Le Couteur DG, Abernethy DR, et al. Reducing drugs in older adults is more. Arch Intern Med 2011;171:868–9.

Ethical Framework for Medication Discontinuation in Nursing Home Residents with Limited Life Expectancy

Jennifer Tjia, MD, MSCE[a],*, Jane Givens, MD, MSCE[b,c]

KEYWORDS

- Ethics • Discontinuation • Medication • End of life
- Nursing home • Dementia

Addressing polypharmacy in the clinical setting requires some acknowledgement of the challenges facing the medication discontinuation process. Anecdotes suggest that many pharmacists and prescribers face barriers to paring down medication regimens. Perhaps the first challenge is recognizing that the concept of "less is more" when applied to medication prescribing is unfamiliar to many clinicians, patients, and families. Although modern day prescription medication use has contributed to improved life expectancy and quality of life for many patients, it is important to acknowledge the evidence documenting preventable harm and unnecessary medication use. Because there are an estimated 1.9 million adverse drug events (ADEs) occurring in US nursing home (NH) residents annually,[1] more than 40% of which are preventable, it is vitally important to discontinue unnecessary medications whenever possible.

In the NH setting, residents use, on average, 7 to 8 medications daily.[2] Many of these medications are inappropriate,[3–5] have been continued beyond their original indication,[6] or contribute to excess medication-related injuries.[1,7,8] Further, many unnecessary medications are used in patients with advanced illness with little expected benefit.[9,10]

It is important for clinicians to be aware of federal regulations germane to the prescribing of unnecessary medications in NH residents (**Box 1**). Specifically, the Nursing Home Reform Act from 1987 (Omnibus Budget Reconciliation Act of 1987

[a] Division of Geriatric Medicine, University of Massachusetts Medical School, 377 Plantation Street, Suite 315, Worcester, MA 01605, USA
[b] Division of Gerontology, Beth Israel Deaconess Medical Center, Boston, MA, USA
[c] Hebrew SeniorLife Institute for Aging Research, 1200 Centre Street, Boston, MA 02131, USA
* Corresponding author.
E-mail address: jennifer.tjia@umassmed.edu

Clin Geriatr Med 28 (2012) 255–272
doi:10.1016/j.cger.2012.01.010
0749-0690/12/$ – see front matter © 2012 Elsevier Inc. All rights reserved.

geriatric.theclinics.com

Box 1
OBRA-87 regulations for unnecessary medications

Unnecessary drugs - (1) General. Each resident's drug regimen must be free from unnecessary drugs. An unnecessary drug is any drug when used:

(i) In excessive dose (including duplicate drug therapy); or

(ii) for excessive duration; or

(iii) without adequate monitoring; or

(iv) without adequate indications for its use; or

(v) in the presence of adverse consequences that indicate the dose should be reduced or discontinued; or

(vi) any combination of the above reasons.

From Omnibus Budget Reconciliation Act of 1987 [OBRA-87]. Public Law No. 100-203. Subtitle C: Nursing Home Reform. F329 Unnecessary drugs. US Congress. Washington DC, 1987.

[OBRA-87])[11] states that "Each resident's drug regimen must be free from unnecessary drugs." The specification put forth in OBRA-87 includes "any drug when used: 1) in excessive dose (including duplicate drug therapy); or 2) for excessive duration; or 3) without adequate monitoring; or 4) without adequate indications for its use; or 5) in the presence of adverse consequences which indicate the dose should be reduced or discontinued; or 6) any combination of the reasons above." These regulations have typically been applied toward Beer's list[3,12] and psychoactive medications. However, a 2006 update to OBRA-87 seeking clarity in the language of what constitute unnecessary medications restated that all medications prescribed to NH residents, not just psychoactive medications, were subject to the same scrutiny and set of administrative guidelines.[13]

Because the primary responsibility of the clinician is to maximize benefit and minimize harm from medical interventions, this article sets forth an ethical framework for medication discontinuation in NH residents with limited life expectancy. This article is organized into 3 sections:

1. Review of ethical principles. Four core ethical principles serve as the basis for medical decision making: beneficence, nonmaleficence, respect for patient autonomy, and justice.
2. How to apply a 4-stage ethical framework to prescribing challenges. This framework considers: (1) medical indication, (2) patient preference, (3) quality of life, and (4) contextual issues. We will present a base case in which the framework is first utilized and 3 cases exemplifying issues arising from conflicts between physicians and family members or surrogate decision makers about prescribing recommendations.
3. Practical considerations for medication discontinuation. This section presents principles for initiating medication review, communicating with patients and families, and executing discontinuation trials.

REVIEW OF ETHICAL PRINCIPLES

There are 4 core ethical principles that serve as the basis for all medical decision making: beneficence, nonmaleficence, respect for patient autonomy, and justice (**Box 2**). The following provides a definition of each and a brief discussion of the relevant issues that apply to NH residents with limited life expectancy.

<blockquote>

Box 2
Four key ethical principles

Beneficence. The concept of beneficence refers to the principle that clinicians should act in the best interest of the patient, typically by determining whether an intervention can fulfill the goals of medicine by providing benefit.

Non-maleficence. Closely related to the imperative of beneficence is the principle of non-maleficence ("first, do no harm"). Practically speaking, this means that clinicians must evaluate the potential risks of initiating, continuing, or discontinuing a medication, in relation to its benefits.

Patient autonomy. The principle of autonomy is defined as the moral right to choose and follow one's own plan of life and action. Respect for autonomy is the moral attitude that disposes one to refrain from interference with the autonomous beliefs and actions of others in the pursuit of their goals.

Justice. Justice is the ethical principle governing the fair and equitable distribution of burdens and benefits to the participants in social institutions. Justice also determines how the rights of various participants are realized within those social institutions. Reform of . . . health policy in accordance with the principles of justice is an ethical imperative, as is the allocation of scare health resources.

From Jonsen A, Siegler M, Winslade W. Clinical ethics. 6th edition New York: McGraw-Hill; 2006.

</blockquote>

Beneficence

The concept of beneficence refers to the principle that clinicians should act in the best interest of the patient, typically by determining whether an intervention (in our case, a medication) can fulfill the goals of medicine by providing benefit.

In the context of NH residents with limited life expectancy, determining whether a medication is beneficial can be complicated. Recent frameworks for prescribing for patients with limited life expectancy[14,15] suggest clinicians consider the act of medication prescribing in terms of several important factors: (1) the patient's prognosis, (2) the initial intention of a therapy, and (3) the time until realizing benefits (or burdens). This holistic approach to prescribing stands in contrast to the more traditional, problem- and guideline-based, medical approach to prescribing that addresses each problem/symptom with a separate medication, typically without regard to life expectancy and time to benefit. The limited life expectancy framework asks the clinician to consider the initial intention of a therapy (ie, the original indication), and explicitly consider whether the indication still exists. For example, if a patient was initially prescribed donepezil for dementia of the Alzheimer's type while residing in the community with mild stage disease, but is currently residing with advanced stage disease in an NH (characterized by a median prognosis of 6 months or less), it can be argued that the original indication for the donepezil (to slow disease progression and forestall NH placement) no longer exists. In this case, the likelihood of clinical benefit is questionable at best.

Nonmaleficence

Closely related to beneficence is the principle of nonmaleficence ("first, do no harm"). Practically speaking, this means that clinicians must evaluate the potential risks of initiating, continuing, or discontinuing a medication, in relation to its benefits.

The spectrum of medication risk can be considered on a range extending from theoretical risk to actual harm. Somewhere in the middle of this spectrum is the burden of drug administration and monitoring with laboratory tests. In the case of a known and indisputable injury attributable to a medication (ie, an ADE), the clinician's risk-benefit equation is relatively simple: the medication should not be recommended to the patient without a compelling reason. However, there are several aspects of NH care that make this more complicated. First, many adverse drug events in this population are clinically unrecognized. At best, these adverse drug events may mimic a new clinical condition, and are often treated with yet another medication in a phenomenon known as a *prescribing cascade*.[16] Perhaps worse, ADEs may be attributed to normal aging (eg, diminished appetite or decreased energy) and contribute to excess and untimely clinical and functional decline. In this situation, the actual risk of harm may be unclear, but the theoretical risk of harm remains very real. Second, many NH residents are cognitively impaired and unable to communicate symptoms indicative of harm. This further reduces the likelihood of recognizing ADEs in this population. For example, many residents with advanced dementia have eating and feeding problems, but it is difficult to discern whether these are attributable to the progression of their disease or to drug-induced nausea or anorexia. Third, the risk of medication discontinuation is often unclear and arguably theoretical because of the lack of relevant studies providing evidence of benefit or harm. Therefore, clinicians considering a medication discontinuation trial are often working with a risk-benefit equation that can seem largely theoretical.

Patient Autonomy

The principle of autonomy is defined as the moral right to choose and follow one's own plan of life and action. Respect for autonomy is the moral attitude that recommends restraint from interfering with the autonomous beliefs and actions of others in the pursuit of their goals.[17]

After weighing the potential benefits and risks of a medical intervention, and making a recommendation to a patient (or proxy decision maker), the patient's preferences about whether to proceed come to the fore. In the NH setting, a common and challenging ethical dilemma facing many physicians is whether the patient's mental capacity, compromised by illness, affects his or her ability to express his or her preferences.[17] Another issue is the difficulty that arises when patient preference creates conflicts, either with the prescriber, or with the wishes of their family.

Justice

The fourth principle is justice. One definition describes justice as "the ethical principle governing the fair and equitable distribution of burdens and benefits to the partici-pants in social institutions."[17] According to this definition, justice determines how the rights of various participants are realized within social institutions and is germane to health policy and the allocation of scarce health resources.

While prescribers are primarily focused on issues at the individual level, attempting to provide appropriate care for particular patients, it is important to consider the greater context of the NH and health care system. Although the growing burden of health care spending is outside the scope of this article, it is helpful to consider that in 2004, the total Medicaid reimbursement for pharmaceuticals used in the NH was $3.3 billion, for an average of 68.3 prescriptions per patient per year, including 6.7 prescriptions per benefit month.[18] It is well known that growing health care expen-ditures are threatening the viability of Medicare in the United States and represent one of the greatest challenges facing health care providers and policy makers to date. ". . . [W]hile it is morally permissible to constrain a person's freely chosen actions only when that person's preferences and actions seriously infringe on the rights and welfare of others,"[17] it can be argued that, at a public health level, the unchecked continuation of medications of questionable benefit to respect patient autonomy (or their family decision makers) creates an ethical challenge for health care systems and health policy makers who grapple with very real challenges of the equitable distribution of limited health care resources.

APPLYING A 4-STAGE ETHICAL FRAMEWORK TO PRESCRIBING CHALLENGES: CLINICIAL CASES
Overview

In *Clinical Ethics*, Jonsen and coworkers[17] suggest a 4-stage approach to organize the relevant facts of a clinical ethical dilemma. Because any number of questions can be asked in a given case, these authors recommend using this rubric to lay out the relevant facts. The 4 topics can be considered as signposts that guide the way through the complexity of the case and are akin to the organizational approach used by clinicians in daily practice. The stages include (1) medical indication, (2) patient preference, (3) quality of life, and (4) contextual issues.

In this section, 4 cases of medication discontinuation are presented: case 1, a base case to illustrate the application of this framework; case 2, a case of decisional conflict between a patient and prescriber; case 3, a case of decisional conflict between a prescriber and surrogate decision maker for a patient lacking decision-making capacity; and case 4, a case of decisional conflict in which a patient or surrogate decision maker requests medication reduction but the prescriber refuses. Each case is followed by an application of the 4-stage framework and then a case synthesis. Note that case 3 includes several variations (scenarios A, B, and C) of conflict that might occur between the patient's and decision maker's preferences.

Case 1 (Base Case)

An 89-year-old woman with diabetes, end-stage renal disease, and multi-infarct dementia is hospitalized with lethargy and decreased oral intake. A urinary tract infection is diagnosed and treated with antibiotics, but the patient has volume depletion and acute-on-chronic renal failure requiring intravenous hydration. Despite therapy, the patient declines, remains oliguric, and becomes unresponsive to voice or noxious stimuli. Administering medications becomes burdensome and difficult, and the physician is asked to change the mode of administration of all medications to either intravenous or per rectum routes. In a family conference, the physician and surrogate decision maker arrive at a consensus that the goal of care is no longer curative or life prolonging but is aimed at providing comfort. The patient is admitted to hospice.

Case analysis

Medical indication. The medical indications in this case include the patient's clinical, functional, and cognitive state; prognosis; and consideration of the current and proposed treatments. Of particular relevance for the therapeutic intervention are the risks, benefits, and probable outcomes for each treatment (in this case, mainly the medications, intravenous fluids, and feeding).[17] For this analysis, the focus remains on the medications.

A summary of this case shows that after initial hospitalization and treatment, the patient's prognosis was poor. The clinician felt that life-prolonging treatments were no longer appropriate, and it was the family's preference to make the goal of care comfort. Hence, the patient was admitted to hospice. Typically, on admission to hospice, a medication review identifies medications aimed at symptom management, and many medications are often discontinued.

Patient preference. Because the patient is unresponsive, surrogate decision makers (typically, family members) work with the clinician to make treatment decisions consistent with patient preferences. If patient preferences are unknown, treatment decisions should be guided by the best interests of the patient. The concept of "best interest" comes from the legal field and can be difficult to apply to health care situations but essentially involves assessing and maximizing the patient's quality of life.

Quality of life. When the goal of care is comfort, quality of life can be considered a life "that is free from avoidable suffering for patients, families and caregivers, in general accordance with the patients' and families' wishes."[19] For this case, maintaining and initiating medications that improve comfort and address symptoms affecting quality of life, such as pain, dyspnea, and secretions, should be prioritized over continuation of medications for primary or secondary prevention and medications to prolong life, particularly if the administration of those medications is burdensome (ie, requiring intravenous administration) or require invasive monitoring (eg, venipunctures). Use of any burdensome medications and medications inconsistent with the goals of care are typically discontinued.

Contextual factors. Contextual factors in this rubric include the social, legal, economic, and institutional circumstances in which the patient care occurs. In this case, the patient was an NH resident whose initial care occurred in the context of a hospital and then in the NH under the auspices of the Medicare hospice benefit. The physician's role in the health care system obligates him or her to provide care to promote and maintain the resident's highest practical mental, physical, and psycho-social well-being, as defined by the resident or representatives,[13] and adhere to federal guidelines about quality prescribing if in the NH setting.[11] Other contextual features in this case include the allocation of scarce health resources (considered under the ethical principal of justice described above) and the influence of religion on clinical decisions. For example, some religions have extensive teachings about health and medical care that may dictate or prohibit certain interventions.

Case synthesis. This case illustrates the application of the analytic framework but involved no ethical conflicts. In this case, the patient was admitted to hospice, and all preventive, curative, and chronic disease medications were discontinued. Medications for symptom relief were used as needed to keep the patient comfortable.

Each of the following cases presents an occurrence of decisional conflict.

Case 2—A Case of Decisional Conflict Between the Patient and the Prescriber

This is a 95-year-old female NH resident with obesity, diabetes mellitus, peripheral vascular disease, chronic kidney disease, anemia, stage IV heart failure, osteoporosis, depression, anxiety, chronic low back pain, chronic headaches, and vertigo. Her medications include glyburide, metformin, cilostazol, lisinopril, alendronate, furosemide, spironolactone, potassium supplement, ferrous sulfate, multivitamin, zinc, vitamin C, vitamin B12 and folate, carisoprodol, butalbital/acetaminophen/caffeine, alprazolam, meclizine, omprazole, and milk of magnesia for constipation. Her medications are reviewed by the prescriber.

On review, the bisphosphonate was started 7 years ago and continued despite evidence that no additional benefit is derived with more than 5 years of treatment.[20] With advanced age, this patient is at high risk of hypoglycemia when treated with glyburide, and the metformin is not indicated in a person with chronic kidney disease and diuretic therapy. Her anxiety may be caused by dyspnea, which is treated with diuretics, but she refused to stop her alprazolam. The patient has also been taking carisoprodol and butalbital/acetaminophen/caffeine for years and is unwilling to stop because she has daily back pain and headaches.

Case analysis
Medical indication. This patient is taking medications of questionable benefit (multivitamin, zinc, vitamin C), some considered inappropriate in elderly patients (alprazolam, carisoprodol, and ferrous sulfate [in certain cases]), one with evidence of overt harm (butalbital/acetaminophen/caffeine causing withdrawal headaches and dependence), some with questionable indications (vitamin B12 and folate, meclizine), and one that has expired its indication (alendronate).

Patient preference. In this case, the patient wants to continue all possible therapy, causing conflict with the recommendations of the prescriber. This presents an ethical challenge. There may be several underlying reasons for this patient's preference. Medications may hold benefit to the patient by symbolizing hope, and a suggestion of discontinuation is, therefore, felt as a loss of hope, abandonment, and concern that the clinician is hastening death. Further, conflict may have arisen because of inadequate communication regarding the patient's underlying concerns. What is in the best interest of the patient in this case is unclear, but some would argue that maintaining trust in the doctor-patient relationship and respecting the patient's values remains paramount.

Quality of life. The patient, already threatened by disease, may need to exert some need for control over her medical management, which may contribute to her overall quality of life. While it may be the clinical opinion of the physician that fewer medications will optimize quality of life, years without apparent harm to date may make this risk more "theoretical" than actual to the patient.

Contextual features. An additional feature of this case is that the NH physician's prescribing is subject to review according to federal standards that call for the patient to be free from unnecessary medications (OBRA 87),[11,13] including numerous explicitly listed inappropriate medications from the Beer's list, such as alprazolam and carisoprodol. This further contributes to the ethical challenge faced by this prescriber.

Case synthesis While the resident has the right to refuse treatment recommendations, the physician should inform the resident about the risks related to the refusal and discuss appropriate alternatives if available. One challenging issue is whether prescribers are obliged to continue prescribing drugs they deem unsafe or unnecessary. Although this is easier to consider when medications are contraindicated or are causing obvious harm, it is more difficult when the drugs are unsafe because of a theoretical risk or if the drug is not causing apparent harm but lacks indication. In these instances, the obligation of the physician is to deliver best quality of care to promote patient welfare.

Another issue is the nature of the prescriber-patient relationship. Some experts would suggest that decisional conflict arises with inadequate communication and that a thorough discussion of the goals of care, prognosis, risks, and benefits of therapy could achieve therapeutic consensus.[21] However, decisional conflict can persist despite the best communication efforts. In such cases, a second clinical opinion (eg, from a clinical subspecialist, palliative care physician, or consultant pharmacist) may be of benefit. Although a consult of an ethics committee is sometimes a consideration in cases of decisional conflict, in practicality, this is usually reserved for medical interventions with greater overt burden (eg, surgical procedures or mechanical ventilation) and not usually used in medication prescribing situations. In this case, the physician should stop medications with overt harm and offer reasonable and safer substitutes where medically indicated. Medications with theoretical risk, but without clear evidence of overt harm, should probably be continued to reflect the patient's preference. The medication regimen should be re-evaluated periodically, particularly at times of new symptom development and acute clinical change.

Case 3—A Case of Decisional Conflict Between the Prescriber and a Surrogate Decision Maker

An 84-year-old female NH resident with advanced dementia, coronary artery disease, type 2 diabetes mellitus, and history of atrial fibrillation (currently in sinus rhythm), is admitted to hospice with a diagnosis of advanced dementia after poor recovery following a bout of recurrent aspiration pneumonia. The patient is totally dependent on others for daily care, spends most of the day in bed, and responds favorably to destimulation therapy. She does not recognize family but appears to enjoy their company during visits. The patient has a good appetite, finishes most meals with assistance, and has no difficulty taking her medications, which include a multivitamin, vitamin C, calcium, vitamin D, fish oil, ferrous sulfate, aspirin, simvastatin, donepezil, memantine, warfarin, metoprolol, oxybutynin, and acetaminophen *as needed*.

Case analysis

Medical indication. On hospice admission, the hospice medical director's medication review results in a consideration to discontinue the donepezil and memantine because their role in advanced dementia is controversial.[22,23] Although there is no clinical trial data showing benefit in this stage of disease, families and clinicians are concerned about acute decline in functional and cognitive status (an adverse drug withdrawal effect) after discontinuation.[24–27] The evidence for such an outcome is currently mixed and based on little data. The multivitamin and vitamin C are also felt to have questionable benefit, as the patient is nutritionally replete,[28] and the warfarin is recommended for discontinuation because venipunctures needed to monitor INR levels are felt to be burdensome.

Patient preference. In a patient without decision making capacity, knowledge of patient preference can be problematic. When known (eg, through an advance directive), the surrogate decision maker should honor the patient's preferences. However, sometimes preferences are unknown. Several scenarios are presented herein based on 3 variations on whether the patient's preference is known and whether the family honors that preference.

  Scenario A: Patient preferences are unknown, and there is a disagreement between clinician and decision-maker. If patient preferences are unknown, the surrogate decision maker must consider the best interests of the patient. This requires that the surrogate's decisions promote the welfare of the patient, which is defined as making choices about relief of suffering, preservation or restoration of function, and quality of life that reasonable persons in similar circumstances are likely to choose.[17] Such choices are often influenced by contextual features such as the family's beliefs and religious views about quality of life and the role of medications in maintaining that life.

  Scenario B: The family wants to continue all medications against the clinician's discontinuation recommendation based on their knowledge of the patient's

preference for aggressive care and an advance directive stating that the patient wants everything possible done. This surrogate is acting in accordance with the patient's preferences. Patient wishes can be known through advance care planning documents, called advance directives, which can take several forms, including surrogate decision making arrangements in the form of living wills.[19] Living will statutes vary across states but generally envision individuals making legally binding arrangements to the effect that they shall not be sustained by medical treatments that artificially prolong the dying process if they are in a terminal condition and can no longer make decisions. The applications of these documents for late-stage disease, in the absence of imminent death, and for the management of chronic disease medications (unless explicitly addressed), can be problematic and illustrate the limitations of these documents in providing practical guidance in real life clinical situations. In the absence of such documentation, evidence of a patient's expressed oral wishes should be sufficient to guide surrogate decision making.

   Scenario C: Even though the patient has always disliked medications and made this known to the doctor, NH staff, and family when possible, the family surrogate decision maker disagrees with the discontinuation recommendations of the clinician. The patient's preferences may be known via previously expressed preferences, but it is possible that a family can disagree with these preferences. Families typically are motivated by the concern that their decision will hasten death and often do not want to take on this responsibility. The family has placed their own self-interest first, and may be hoping to make life last as long as possible. It is often difficult for families to let go, and this may lead to decisions inconsistent with goals of care and patient preferences.

Quality of life. Although perceptions about quality of life are arguably personal and influenced by worldviews and religious perspective, measures from the medical literature highlight important burdens to the patient associated with medication administration, particularly in patients with cognitive impairment and functional limitations. For example, oral and feeding problems, either from apraxia or other causes, develop in many patients with advanced dementia, which makes the daily oral administration of multiple medications challenging. Further, polypharmacy can exacerbate feeding problems by causing anorexia attributable to the pill burden alone. In other cases, appropriate monitoring of medications requires repeated venipuncture (eg, warfarin) that may be perceived by cognitively impaired patients as invasive and intrusive.[29] Finally, undiagnosed side effects of medications may result in poor quality of life by contributing to symptoms such as lightheadedness, nausea, or weakness. Unfortunately, many of these symptoms are often inappropriately attributed to old age itself in a practice coined *ageism* by the National Institute of Aging's first director, Dr Robert Butler.[30] That said, the physician's perception of quality of life may reflect values of the dominant medical culture that are not shared by all, including the patient or family. It is important for providers to refrain from imposing their values on patients with limited life expectancy and their families. "A humane care system is one that people can trust to serve them well as they die, even if their needs and beliefs call for departures from practices or idealized expectations of caregivers."[19]

Contextual features. Hospice is paying for the medications, and it may appear to the family that the hospice providers have a financial interest in stopping medications. Insistence on stopping medications against the wishes of the family can undermine the relationship between the family and hospice and may cause the family distress

Table 1
Barriers to medication discontinuation

Patient/Family Barriers	Prescriber Barriers
Feeling of abandonment	Prescribed by another physician
Medications represent hope	No evidence to guide discontinuation
Fear of causing patient death	"Ageism" – Adverse drug effect is masquerading as a symptom felt to be common to aging[30] No guidelines Perception of little or no reimbursement for time of medication review and family discussion

and concern that may detract from the goal of providing comfort to the patient and family.

Case synthesis. Scenario A. When the patient's wishes are unknown, and the clinician recommends medication discontinuation, but the surrogate decision maker is not in agreement, it is likely wise to maintain medications as prescribed and readdress with changes in clinical status, while trying to elicit the family's underlying values for decision making.

Scenario B. In this case, with an advance directive favoring medication use, the clinician should maintain medications as prescribed and readdress with changes in clinical status while respecting the family's goals of care. This may place the physician in conflict with obligations to minimize therapy with little or minimal benefit in the setting of limited clinical resources, behind the welfare of the patient and their values.

Scenario C. Although case precedent has shown that courts will side with patient preferences over family wishes in situations of conflict, such as in famous cases such as Terry Schiavo, most instances of chronic disease medication discontinuation are less contentious. Clinicians typically accede to the surrogate decision-maker wishes in these cases. It may be helpful to understand whether a surrogate's decision is influenced by a particular religious view of life and clinical care. Discussions may reveal that the medications symbolize hope and that discontinuation represents loss of hope and feeling of abandonment. There may be issues unknown to the prescriber such as unresolved issues/guilt/need for family reconciliation, or internal family disagreement. Finally, lack of trust in the NH or physician may compel family to assume the role of vigilant caregiver, which may manifest as continuing all care against prescriber advice (**Table 1**).

There may be a role of an ethics committee in this case if available. Many hospitals and health care institutions have used ethics consultants to addresses problematic cases. "The goal of ethics consultation is to improve the process and outcome of care by identifying, analyzing, and working to resolve ethical problems encountered in individual cases. To achieve this goal, it is necessary to identify the issue that precipitated the consultation and to facilitate resolution through patient and staff education and the opportunity for informed and respectful discussion of the problem. Consultation also may help deeply involved parties see cases in different perspectives."[17]

Case 4—A Case of Decisional Conflict in which a Patient or Surrogate Decision Maker Requests Medication Reduction but the Prescriber Refuses

A 90-year-old female NH resident with coronary artery disease and atrial fibrillation (not on warfarin because of fall risk) feels she takes too many medications and thinks they contribute to her weakness and anorexia. She is on metoprolol, furosemide, lisinopril, aspirin, fish oil, gemfibrozil, digoxin and atorvastatin. The NH doctor has prescribed mirtazapine for depression and anorexia. The patient and family ask to review and stop any unnecessary medications, but the NH doctor says "I don't have time and I can't take the risk—the cardiologist prescribed them." The family read about her medications on the internet, and learned that digoxin can cause many side effects and needs to be monitored. They ask for digoxin level to be checked. The level is 1.7 μg/mL; the family is told this is within normal limits and that no changes are necessary.

Case analysis

Medical indication. It is important to remember that "therapeutic" levels of digoxin can still cause side effects and may be contributing to the patient's anorexia. Further, the indication for digoxin in this case is controversial; digoxin is not first-line treatment for rate control in atrial fibrillation, and her heart rate may already be controlled with metoprolol. Additionally, the combination of atorvastatin and gemfibrozil in this patient increases the patient's risk for myopathy. Although her NH doctor has treated her anorexia with mirtazapine, both for presumed depression and loss of appetite, another explanation is that the anorexia is caused by the digoxin, the weakness is caused by the combination of antihypertensives, and the use of mirtazapine represents a "prescribing cascade," whereby the side effects of the initial medications are misdiagnosed as symptoms of another problem, resulting in further prescribing. This is a pharmacologic example of a feedback loop.

Patient preference. The patient's preference in this case is to take fewer medications. The physician's reluctance to review and discontinue medications may result in the continuation of unwanted and unnecessary medical treatments, which can contribute to less-than-optimal care in the face of limited life expectancy, according to the Institute of Medicine's definition of a quality death.[19] More concerning, it is important to recall that "Anglo-American law starts with the premise of thoroughgoing self-determining," which includes the right of individuals to refuse medical treatments.[19]

Quality of life. The physician's refusal to discontinue or review medications can be considered an example of dishonoring the patient's values and wishes, which can further detract from the patient's quality of life and the trust in the doctor-patient relationship.

Contextual feature. Again, the NH physician is subject to the OBRA-87 regulations stating that patients should be free of unnecessary medications. However, in this case, the art of medicine makes the identification of these medications quite challenging. Further, it takes time to review these medications and coordinate care with outside consultants (ie, the cardiologist). Although the physician may feel that there is insufficient time and compensation for this activity, such a clinical encounter is actually a highly complex medical decision that can be appropriately compensated by Medicare in the United States with appropriate documentation.

Further barriers to clinician discontinuation are not insignificant. Many prescriber may be unaware of tools or evidence to guide "deprescribing."[21,31] Or, a clinician may feel that he or she lacks the necessary skill set. In the end, the clinician invokes the use of their "best clinical judgment," and often clinical inertia leads to the continuation of medications without adequate indication or monitoring.

Case synthesis. Over the years, the elderly patient can accumulate a regimen of many drugs from many providers. A thorough reassessment of every medication in the regimen can be undertaken to identify medications eligible for discontinuation trial. Although pharmacists are typically considered central to medication regimen reviews, the attending physician plays a key leadership role in medication management by developing, monitoring, and modifying the medication regimen in conjunction with residents, pharmacists, and direct care staff.[13] As such, physicians should be both receptive to pharmacist review recommendations and capable of conducting medication reviews themselves to identify harmful and questionably beneficial medications. Good clinical practice and US federal regulations call for periodic medication regimen reviews.[6]

PRACTICAL ISSUES

Although there are rubrics to guide the appropriate initiation of a prescription medication, equivalent approaches to deprescribing have only recently emerged and are not widely known. "Although some practitioners advocate keeping a 'time-tested' regimen intact even if the validity of its original indications is obscure, we take a different view on the risks and benefits involved. A patient taking a medication without a clear ongoing indication for its use remains at risk for all potential toxicities without deriving any benefit."[6]

When to Conduct a Medication Review for Potential Discontinuation

A medication regimen review, as defined in the federal regulations, is a thorough evaluation of the medication regimen with the goal of promoting positive outcomes and minimizing adverse consequences associated with medication.[13] There are numerous opportunities for medication review in NH residents with limited life expectancy, including NH admission, readmission after hospitalization, serious change in condition, polypharmacy (eg, taking 10 or more daily medications), difficulty taking medications by mouth, persistent nausea or early satiety, burden of drug cost, patient or family dislike of polypharmacy, or entry to hospice.

On NH admission, some medications that may have been beneficial in the community (eg, acetylcholinesterase inhibitors to forestall NH placement) may no longer be indicated or may have regulatory constraints (eg, atypical antipsychotic medications for behavior management in dementia). Some residents may be admitted on medications for an undocumented chronic condition or without a clear indication as to why a medication was begun or should be continued.[13] Further, many residents entering from the community have been nonadherent to long-term medications; the diligent dispensing of all such medications on NH admission can result in toxicity in patients who had been substantially nonadherent.[6] It is expected that the attending physician and NH staff determine if continuing the medications is justified.[13]

The need for review is equally heightened for residents readmitted to the NH from the hospital, where additional medications may have been added to treat acute problems that may not persist beyond the hospital stay,[6] such as proton pump inhibitors for gastrointestinal prophylaxis. Preliminary evidence suggests that hospitalization is associated with increased use of unnecessary medications in NH residents.[9] Once the acute phase has stabilized, the prescriber should consider whether medications are still relevant.[13]

Review is also warranted when the patient has a serious change in condition, including an unexpected clinical problem or decline. The federal guidelines suggest that the potential contribution of the medication regimen to an unanticipated decline or newly emerging or worsening symptoms needs to be recognized and evaluated, and the regimen modified when appropriate.[13] One specific example is the development of new eating or feeding problems that may represent a new ADE. In addition, polypharmacy itself is a risk factor for ADEs and is itself a reasonable indication for medication review. And, upon entry to hospice, medications should again be reviewed for appropriateness and consistency with goals of care.

A Patient-Centered Approach to Performing a Systematic Medication Review

A stepwise approach to medication review builds on Holmes' criteria for prescribing in limited life expectancy,[15] including (1) reviewing patient goals of care, (2) understanding patient prognosis, (3) understanding medication indication/treatment target, and (4) assessing current or previous injury from medications. Each of these steps is consistent with OBRA-87 guidance about reviewing and documenting indications for the use of each medication in the NH.[13]

Goals of care

Regardless of diagnosis, the patient (or family's) goals of care may be life prolongation regardless of the quality of life, remaining symptom free (maximizing symptom-free survival), remaining functionally or cognitively intact as long as possible, or remaining comfortable. This is consistent with OBRA-87 guidance recommending that each resident's goals and preferences be considered when evaluating the indications of medication use.[13]

Patient prognosis

There should also be recognition of the need for end-of-life or palliative care.[13] Despite the well-documented challenges in prognosticating life expectancy, there are some guides that may be helpful to clinicians, patients, and their families in this endeavor. For example, certain types of aggressive cancer (eg, pancreatic cancer, small cell lung cancer, and malignant melanomas) are generally associated with poor prognoses. Noncancer conditions associated with poor prognoses include stage IV heart failure and advanced dementia. The presence of one of these conditions may help contextualize the overall clinical situation for the patient and the family.

Further, although life expectancy is the most prominent feature of prognosis, prognoses may also include qualitative assessments of the likely physical and mental course of a person's illness to death. Planning can be affected by prospects of physical disability, intolerable symptoms (such as persistent nausea or weakness), or mental dysfunction.[19]

Indication/treatment target

It is helpful to characterize the indication and treatment target for each medication the patient is prescribed. Some medications are clearly necessary, such as those for acute symptom management of pain. However, other medications for secondary prevention (ie, to prevent recurrent events), such as statins after a myocardial infarction, or primary prevention (ie, prevention of conditions that have not occurred), such as tamoxifen for the prevention of breast cancer or bisphosphonates for vertebral or hip fractures, may not be indicated. A systematic review of the indication for each medication, considered in light of the resident's goals of care and response to treatment (including progress or lack of progress toward the therapeutic goal), will help to inform a benefit-risk equation that may identify medications no longer indicated. Whether the intended or actual benefit is sufficient to justify the potential risk or adverse consequences associated with a selected medication, dose, and duration should be documented in the medical record.[13]

Assessment of current or previous drug injury

It is useful to consider whether any of the medications have already contributed to harm. In addition to more obvious injuries, such as bleeding, rash, or allergic reaction, clinicians should be aware that injury may be anorexia, nausea, orthostatic hypotension, or generalized weakness. We suggest that it is not enough to assume that all is well if the patient is not complaining, particularly because this population may have trouble communicating and may have adverse drug events misinterpreted as a new symptom requiring drug therapy (recall "prescribing cascades"). A common geriatric pearl from Dr Jerry Avorn suggests that "any new symptom in an elderly patient should be considered a drug side effect until proven otherwise". The OBRA-87 regulations have operationalized this pearl in their official guidance: "the potential contribution of the medication regimen to an unanticipated decline or newly emerging or worsening symptom [should be] recognized and evaluated, and the regimen modified when appropriate."[13] Such information may help to prioritize medications to be discontinued, with highest priority given to drugs causing adverse effects.

How to Execute a Discontinuation Trial

A stepwise approach to discontinuation is described in detail by Bain and coworkers[31] and Woodward.[21] Briefly, a formalized approach after the decision has been made to recommend a discontinuation trial is to: plan; communicate; coordinate with the patient, family, and other clinicians (including nurses); and to monitor for beneficial or harmful effects.

Discussions with the patient and family

Deprescribing should be considered in partnership with patient and family (**Box 3**). The patient and caregiver should be informed of the purpose (or lack of purpose) of each medication, the likely current adverse effects, and medication risks. Drugs to be discontinued, substituted, or reduced can be prioritized, with preference given to drugs causing adverse effects, drugs without indication, drugs used for primary prevention, drugs for secondary prevention. Families may help in prioritizing and identifying problematic medications. For example, a study by Jachuck and colleagues[32] suggests that family members are most likely to report drug side effects, even more than the patients themselves, whereas physicians are least likely to detect a patient's medication side effects. The suggested deprescribing regimen should be the agreed upon, incorporating patient priorities. As with any intervention, a presentation of the indications/risks/benefits should be presented, followed by a plan for monitoring and what to expect, including a plan to revisit and re-review.

Plan, coordinate, and communicate

From a clinical and health system perspective, deprescribing should be undertaken as a team approach, involving the prescriber, pharmacist, and nursing staff.[21] The prescriber should contact other members of the team to ensure that all are aware of the plan and in agreement with the overall process. For example, if a prescriber initiates an antipsychotic taper trial without coordination with nursing staff, and a patient experiences recurrence of hallucinations or challenging behaviors in the subsequent days, a covering physician may embark on a major medical workup and enlist psychiatric evaluation in lieu of restarting the medication. This may drain resources and lead to unintended consequences such as inappropriate antibiotic treatment for a questionable urinalysis result. Team coordination and communication will increase patient safety, help put nonpharmacologic approaches to resident conditions in place when appropriate, and can increase the probability of success with tapering trials.

Box 3
Communicating with families

Assessments Needed in Devising Medication Review in Limited Life Expectancy

Disease status and symptom assessment

- What are the diagnosis and the prognosis?
- How is the disease likely to affect the patient?
- What other current physical or emotional problems are relevant?
- What symptoms are present, and what symptoms are likely to emerge?

Preferences and goals

- Have patient and family preferences, beliefs, and goals been discussed?
- Has a surrogate decision maker been identified if the patient becomes unable to participate in decisions?

Therapy review and evaluation

- What medications are being used and with what results? What potential drug interactions require monitoring?
- On the basis of patient status, should medications be continued, adjusted, or discontinued?
- What nonpharmacologic therapies are being used or should be considered?
- What health care providers are involved in patient care?
- What are the benefits and burdens (for patient, family, and caregivers) of the therapies being provided, and what are the alternatives?

Adapted from Field M, Cassell C. Institute of Medicine Report. Approaching death: improving care at the end of life. Washington DC: National Academy Press; 1997.

Monitor

Bain suggests a gradual dose reduction for certain medications, including all psychopharmacologic medications. This process involves a stepwise tapering of a dose to determine whether symptoms, conditions, or risks can be managed using a lower dose or whether the medication can be discontinued. However, particularly with psychoactive medications, it is important to consider whether there is a risk of adverse drug withdrawal events (defined as a clinically significant set of symptoms or signs cause by the removal of a drug). Most medications should be tapered over the course of days to weeks, particularly those used on a long-term basis. In some cases, such as for antipsychotic medications, there is evidence from clinical trials[33–35] that this gradual taper approach can result in sustained discontinuation without exacerbation of patient symptoms. Drugs without known adverse drug withdrawal effects, such as proton pump inhibitors, can be discontinued abruptly **(Table 2)**.

SUMMARY

A recent editorial by health economist Victor Fuchs summarized the current challenges with health care delivery in this way: "Most physicians want to deliver 'appropriate' care. Most want to practice 'ethically', but it is difficult to know what is 'appropriate' and what is 'ethical'."[36] This characterization is particularly true for medication use and deprescribing in elderly NH residents with limited life expectancy. Medical ethics sets 4 key principles (beneficence, nonmaleficence, patient autonomy, and justice) to guide practice. However, decisional conflicts will

Table 2
Medications commonly associated with adverse drug withdrawal events

Medication	Type of Withdrawal Reaction	Withdrawal Event
Alpha-antagonist antihypertensive	P	Agitation, headache, hypertension, palpitations
Angiotensin-converting enzyme inhibitor	P,D	Heart failure, hypertension
Antianginal	D	Angina pectoris (myocardial ischemia)
Anticonvulsant	P,D	Anxiety, depression, seizures
Antidepressant	P,D	Akathisia, anxiety, chills, coryza, gastrointestinal distress, headache, insomnia, irritability, malaise, myalgia, recurrence of depression
Anti-Parkinson agent	P,D,N	Hypotension, psychosis, pulmonary embolism, rigidity, tremor
Antipsychotic	P	Dyskinesias, insomnia, nausea, restlessness
Baclofen	P,N	Agitation, anxiety, confusion, depression, hallucinations, hypertonia, insomnia, mania, nightmares, paranoia, seizures
Benzodiazepine	P	Agitation, anxiety, confusion, delirium, insomnia, seizures
Beta-blocker	P,D	Angina pectoris, anxiety, hypertension, myocardial infarction, tachycardia
Corticosteroid	P,N	Anorexia, hypotension, nausea, weakness
Digoxin	D	Heart failure, palpitations
Diuretic	D	Heart failure, hypertension
Histamine-2 blocker	D	Recurrence of esophagitis and indigestion symptoms
Narcotic analgesic	P	Abdominal cramping, anger, anxiety, chills, diaphoresis, diarrhea, insomnia, restlessness
Nonsteroidal anti-inflammatory drug	D	Recurrence of arthritis and gout symptoms
Sedative or hypnotic (eg, barbiturate)	P	Anxiety, dizziness, muscle twitches, tremor
Statin	D,N	Cardiogenic shock, early neurological deterioration, heart failure, myocardial infarction, ventricular arrhythmia

Abbreviations: D, exacerbation of underlying condition; N, new set of symptoms; P, physiological withdrawal.
From Bain KT, Holmes HM, Beers MH, et al. Discontinuing medications: a novel approach for revising the prescribing stage of the medication-use process. J Am Geriatr Soc 2008;56(10):1946–52.

continue between providers and patients, and physicians will continue to struggle with the dilemma of balancing the primacy of patient welfare, values, and beliefs against the desire for promising, but often minimally beneficial and harmful, medications that threaten limited clinical resources. Despite these challenges, physicians should be able to perform systematic medication reviews and monitor discontinuation trials in their NH patients for whom this is consistent with their goals of care.

REFERENCES

1. Gurwitz JH, Field TS, Judge J, et al. The incidence of adverse drug events in two large academic long-term care facilities. Am J Med 2005;118(3):251–8.
2. Doshi JA, Shaffer T, Briesacher BA. National estimates of medication use in nursing homes: findings from the 1997 Medicare Current Beneficiary Survey and the 1996 Medical Expenditure Survey. J Am Geriatr Soc 2005;53(3):438–43.
3. Beers MH, Ouslander JG, Rollingher I, et al. Explicit criteria for determining inappropriate medication use in nursing home residents. UCLA Division of Geriatric Medicine. Arch Int Med 1991;151(9):1825–32.
4. Beers MH, Ouslander JG, Fingold SF, et al. Inappropriate medication prescribing in skilled-nursing facilities. Ann Intern Med 1992;117(8):684–9.
5. Perri M 3rd, Menon AM, Deshpande AD, et al. Adverse outcomes associated with inappropriate drug use in nursing homes. Ann Pharmacother 2005;39(3):405–11.
6. Avorn J, Gurwitz JH. Drug use in the nursing home. Ann Intern Med 1995;123(3):195–204.
7. Field TS, Gurwitz JH, Avorn J, et al. Risk factors for adverse drug events among nursing home residents. Arch Intern Med 2001;161(13):1629–34.
8. Lau DT, Kasper JD, Potter DEB, et al. Hospitalization and Death Associated With Potentially Inappropriate Medication Prescriptions Among Elderly Nursing Home Residents. Arch Intern Med 2005;165(1):68–74.
9. Tjia J, Rothman MR, Kiely DK, et al. Daily medication use in nursing home residents with advanced dementia. J Am Geriatr Soc 2010;58(5):880–8.
10. Riechelmann RP, Krzyzanowska MK, Zimmermann C. Futile medication use in terminally ill cancer patients. Support Care Cancer 2009;17(6):745–8.
11. Omnibus Budget Reconciliation Act of 1987 [OBRA-87]. Public Law No. 100-203. Subtitle C: Nursing Home Reform. F329 Unnecessary drugs. US Congress. Washington DC, 1987.
12. Beers MH. Explicit criteria for determining potentially inappropriate medication use by the elderly. An update. Arch Intern Med 1997;157(14):1531–6.
13. Centers for Medicare and Medicaid Services. Transmittal 22. (December 15 2006.) Available at: http://www.cms.hhs.gov/transmittals/downloads/R22SOMA.pdf. Accessed October 17, 2011.
14. Stevenson JP, Currow DC, Abernethy AP. Frameworks for prescribing in comorbid illness. J Pain Symptom Manage 2007;34(2):117–8.
15. Holmes HM, Hayley DC, Alexander GC, et al. Reconsidering medication appropriateness for patients late in life. Arch Intern Med 2006;166(6):605–9.
16. Rochon PA, Gurwitz JH. Optimising drug treatment for elderly people: the prescribing cascade. BMJ 1997;315(7115):1096–9.
17. Jonsen A, Siegler M, Winslade W. Clinical Ethics. 6th ed. New York: McGraw-Hill; 2006.
18. Mathematica Policy Research. Chartbook: Medicaid Pharmacy Benefit Use and Reimbursement in 2004. Available at: https://www.cms.gov/MedicaidDataSources GenInfo/downloads/Pharmacy_Rx_Chartbook_2004.pdf. Accessed October 25, 2011.
19. Field M, Cassell C. Institute of Medicine Report. Approaching death: improving care at the end of life. Washington DC: National Academy Press; 1997.
20. Black DM, Schwartz AV, Ensrud KE, et al. Effects of continuing or stopping alendronate after 5 years of treatment: the Fracture Intervention Trial Long-term Extension (FLEX): a randomized trial. JAMA 2006;296(24):2927–38.

21. Woodward M. Deprescribing: achieving better health outcomes for older people through reducing medications. J Pharm Pract Res 2003;33:323–8.
22. Parsons C, Hughes CM, Passmore AP, et al. Withholding, discontinuing and withdrawing medications in dementia patients at the end of life: a neglected problem in the disadvantaged dying? Drugs Aging 2010;27(6):435–49.
23. Parsons C, Briesacher BA, Givens JL, et al. Cholinesterase inhibitor and memantine use in newly admitted nursing home residents with dementia. J Am Geriatr Soc 2011;59(7):1253–9.
24. Fillit H, Hofbauer RK, Setyawan J, et al. Memantine discontinuation and the health status of nursing home residents with Alzheimer's disease. J Am Med Dir Assoc 2010;11:636–44.
25. Daiello LA, Ott BR, Lapane KL, et al. Effect of discontinuing cholinesterase inhibitor therapy on behavioral and mood symptoms in nursing home patients with dementia. Am J Geriatr Pharmacother 2009;7:74–83.
26. Rainer M, Mucke HAM, Krüger-Rainer C, et al. Cognitive relapse after discontinuation of drug therapy in Alzheimer's disease: cholinesterase inhibitors versus nootropics. J Neural Transm 2001;108:1327–33.
27. Lee J, Monette J, Sourial N, et al. The use of a cholinesterase inhibitor review committee in long-term care. J Am Med Dir Assoc 2007;8:243–7.
28. Huang H-Y, Caballero B, Chang S, et al. The Efficacy and safety of multivitamin and mineral supplement use to prevent cancer and chronic disease in adults: a systematic review for a national institutes of health state-of-the-science conference. Ann Int Med 2006;145(5):372–85.
29. Brauner DJ, Muir JC, Sachs GA. Treating nondementia illnesses in patients with dementia. JAMA 2000;283(24):3230–5.
30. Butler RN. Ageism in America. The Anti-Ageism Taskforce at the International Longevity Center. Available at: http://www.graypanthersmetrodetroit.org/Ageism_In_America_-_ILC_Book_2006.pdf. Accessed October 26, 2011.
31. Bain KT, Holmes HM, Beers MH, et al. Discontinuing medications: a novel approach for revising the prescribing stage of the medication-use process. J Am Geriatr Soc 2008;56(10):1946–52.
32. Jachuck SJ, Brierley H, Jachuck S, et al. The effect of hypotensive drugs on the quality of life. J R Coll Gen Pract 1982;32(235):103–5.
33. Ray WA, Taylor JA, Meador KG, et al. Reducing antipsychotic drug use in nursing homes. A controlled trial of provider education. Arch Intern Med 1993;153(6):713–21.
34. Bridges-Parlet S, Knopman D, Steffes S. Withdrawal of neuroleptic medications from institutionalized dementia patients: results of a double-blind, baseline-treatment-controlled pilot study. J Geriatr Psychiatry Neurol 1997;10(3):119–26.
35. Findlay DJ, Sharma J, McEwen J, et al. Double-blind controlled withdrawal of thioridazine treatment in elderly female inpatients with senile dementia. Int J Ger Psych 1989;4(2):115–20.
36. Fuchs VR. The doctor's dilemma—what is "appropriate" care? N Engl J Med 2011; 365(7):585–7.

Pharmacokinetics and Pharmacodynamic Changes Associated with Aging and Implications for Drug Therapy

Leah Church Sera, PharmD*, Mary Lynn McPherson, PharmD, BCPS, CPE

KEYWORDS
- Pharmacokinetics • Pharmacodynamics • Aging • Elderly
- Polypharmacy • Drug therapy

The population of older adults in the United States continues to expand, and the percentage of patients with multiple comorbid disease states and complex drug regimens has increased as well. The National Center for Health Statistics reported that the percentage of patients age 65 and older taking 3 or more prescription drugs increased from 38% from 1988 to 1994 to 65% from 2005 to 2008.[1] Nearly 20% of patients in this age group take at least 10 medications in any given week.[2] Knowledge of the physiologic changes associated with aging is vital to providing optimal pharmaceutical care to geriatric patients.

The process of aging is associated with multiple biological mechanisms. These include damage to mitochondrial and nuclear DNA caused by increased oxidative stress, increased lipid peroxidation, telomere shortening, altered gene expression, and upregulation of cell apoptosis.[3–5] Ultimately, these mechanisms result in changes in body composition and organ function, which alter both the pharmacokinetics and pharmacodynamics of drugs.

Managing drug therapy in elderly patients is often problematic, because there is a lack of evidence on which to base prescribing decisions. Many randomized, controlled trials exclude older patients, and even trials specifically conducted in geriatric populations may include only relatively healthy subjects.[6] Drugs often are prescribed for older patients at lower doses than normally prescribed for younger individuals because of concern about reduced elimination, multiple comorbidities, and the potential for drug-drug interactions.[7] However, in many cases, these dose

Department of Pharmacy Practice and Science, University of Maryland School of Pharmacy, Baltimore, MD 21201, USA
* Corresponding author.
E-mail address: lsera@rx.umaryland.edu

Clin Geriatr Med 28 (2012) 273–286
doi:10.1016/j.cger.2012.01.007
0749-0690/12/$ – see front matter © 2012 Elsevier Inc. All rights reserved.

Table 1
Pharmacokinetic changes in the elderly

Process	Effect on Drug Disposition

Absorption	• Possibly reduced intestinal absorption of agents requiring active transport
	• Reduced first-pass metabolism
	  ○ Increased absorption of some high-clearance drugs
	  ○ Decreased absorption of drugs from prodrugs

Distribution	• Altered free fraction of some drugs
	  ○ Increased free fraction of albumin-bound drugs
	  ○ Decreased free fraction of α 1-glycoprotein-bound drugs
	• Altered volume of distribution
	  ○ Increased half-life for lipophilic drugs
	• Increased permeability of blood-brain barrier

Metabolism	• Delayed metabolism of high clearance drugs
Excretion	• Increased half-life for water-soluble drugs

Adapted from Corsonello A, Pedone C, Antonelli Incalzi R. Age-related pharmacokinetic and pharmacodynamic changes and related risk of adverse drug reactions. Curr Med Chem 2010;17: 571–84 and Shi S, Morike K, Klotz U. The clinical implications of ageing for rational drug therapy. Eur J Clin Pharmacol 2008;64:183–99.

adjustments are empiric and may potentially result in subtherapeutic outcomes. The complex drug regimens of many elderly patients, along with altered pharmacokinetics and pharmacodynamics of many drugs, means that the potential for adverse drug reactions is increased in this population.

PHARMACOKINETICS

Pharmacokinetics refers to the disposition of a drug in the body. The absorption, distribution, metabolism, and excretion of medications are affected to varying extents by the normal aging process and by disease states commonly associated with increasing age. Common age-related alterations in pharmacokinetics are summarized in **Table 1**.

ABSORPTION

Of the 4 pharmacokinetic parameters to be discussed, absorption appears to be the least affected by the natural changes that occur with age. The absorption of drugs into the systemic circulation may occur via the gut, as with oral preparations, or via the skin, muscle, subcutaneous layer, or lungs.

The bioavailability of a drug refers to the portion of a dose that reaches the systemic circulation. Intravenously administered medications have bioavailability of 100%, whereas the bioavailability of drugs administered orally depends on the extent of absorption in the gut and first-pass metabolism.[8] The bioavailability of some medications and nutrients may be altered in older patients because of changes in the gut and liver.

Oral Administration

There are several physiologic changes that occur in the aging gastrointestinal tract, including reduction in intestinal blood flow[9] as well as decreased gut motility and delayed gastric emptying caused by a loss of local neural control.[10] Gastric acid production may be reduced, although this may be caused by atrophic gastritis that frequently occurs in old age rather than a natural aging process. There is evidence that the active diffusion of some nutrients, such as iron, calcium, and vitamin B12 is diminished[11]; however, most drugs are absorbed passively and appear not to be affected. For instance, studies on the absorption of penicillin, diazepam, lorazepam, metronidazole, and indomethacin in the elderly have shown no difference compared with the absorption in younger subjects.[12] The use of drugs that slow or inhibit gastrointestinal motility are likely to have a more pronounced effect on absorption than physiologic alterations.[13]

First-pass metabolism occurs within the gut for substrates of cytochrome P450 3A4 and P-glycoprotein[4] as well as within the liver. Reduction of the first-pass effect caused by diminished liver mass and blood flow[14] may affect the extent of absorption for drugs of high clearance because of a reduction in first-pass metabolism. The hepatic extraction ratio is a measure of the liver's ability to eliminate drugs from systemic circulation; drugs with high extraction ratios may be cleared during a single pass, whereas drugs with low extraction ratios are not as efficiently eliminated. Labetalol, nifedipine, and verapamil showed increased absorption in the elderly; however, other high-extraction drugs showed no difference in oral bioavailability.[15] Drugs that require enzymatic conversion to the active drug moiety, such as the case of enalapril (a pro-drug) being converted to enalaprilat (the pharmacologically active entity), will have a lower serum level with a reduction in first pass effect.[16]

Other Routes of Administration

Other routes of drug absorption may also be affected by the aging process. Reduction of tissue blood perfusion may decrease the rate of absorption of subcutaneous or intramuscular administration of drugs.[13] Decreased absorption via the inhaled route may occur in the elderly because of reductions in chest wall compliance, ventilation-perfusion matching, and alveolar surface area.[18] Additionally, many older patients may have difficulty using inhalation devices appropriately because of age-related changes in dexterity and disease states such as osteoarthritis and Parkinson's disease.[19] Transdermal drug delivery avoids issues associated with first-pass metabolism. There is an age-related reduction in the hydration and lipophilic content of older skin, which may theoretically reduce the absorption of hydrophilic drugs; however, no significant differences in transdermal absorption between young and elderly patients have been seen in clinical practice.[20]

DISTRIBUTION

The distribution of a drug is primarily dependent on its volume of distribution and the extent of protein binding, both of which may be affected by the aging process.

Protein Binding

The 2 primary drug binding proteins are α-1-acid glycoprotein and albumin. Increases in α-1-acid glycoprotein are seen in many age-related disorders such as cancer and inflammatory disease and may decrease the pharmacologically active free fraction of lidocaine, propranolol, and other basic drugs.[21] Albumin levels are on average 20% lower in elderly patients, which may increase the free fraction of acidic drugs such as naproxen, phenytoin, and warfarin.[21,22] However, there appears to be little change in the area under the curve (AUC) for most drugs.[4] AUC represents the extent of drug exposure in the body. Small increases in AUC may be expected from intravenously administered drugs with a high hepatic extraction ratio and extensive protein binding (**Table 2**).[23]

Table 2
Selected drugs significantly bound to plasma proteins[21,59]

Plasma Protein	Drug	Protein Binding (%)
Albumin (acidic drugs)	Naproxen	99
	Phenytoin	95
	Tolbutamide	95
	Warfarin	99
A 1-glycoprotein (basic drugs)	Lidocaine	80
	Propranolol	90
	Quinidine	88
	Imipramine	89

Volume of Distribution

Volume of distribution is a term used to describe the ratio of total drug in the body to the amount of drug in plasma. Changes in body composition that may alter volume of distribution in elderly patients include a decrease in total body water and an increase in fat content.[24] The volume of distribution of hydrophilic drugs decreases with aging with a consequent increase in drug concentration, whereas the opposite is true for lipophilic drugs (**Table 3**). The plasma half-life of a drug is directly related to volume of distribution; if the volume of distribution increases, as with lipophilic agents, the drug is retained longer in the body.[13] Decreased muscle mass evident in older patients may also affect volume of distribution. Drugs that are active in muscle tissue, such as digoxin, may have a decreased volume of distribution and increased plasma concentrations, potentially leading to digoxin toxicity.[25]

P-Glycoprotein

P-glycoprotein (P-gp) is a membrane-associated protein located in many tissues, including the gut-kidney and blood-brain barrier, whose primary function is as an efflux pump for xenobiotics.[25] A study of duodenal P-gp activity in older and younger patients suggested no appreciable difference in P-gp activity. However, a study involving the P-gp substrate, verapamil, showed decreased P-gp activity in the

Table 3
Selected lipophilic and hydrophilic drugs[13]

Drug	Effect of Age
Hydrophilic	Volume of distribution decreases
Ethanol	Plasma concentration increases
Cimetidine	Half-life decreases
Digoxin	
Levodopa	
Morphine	
Propicillin	
Lipophilic	Volume of distribution increases
Thiopental	Plasma concentration decreases
Amitriptyline	Half-life increases
Diazepam	
Clomethiazole	
Tolbutamide	

blood-brain barriers of older subjects,[26] which could indicate that the aging brain is at higher risk for drug exposure. P-gp activity in elderly patients has not been extensively studied; the risk of toxicity related to alterations in P-gp expression in tissues other than the blood-brain barrier is as yet unknown.

METABOLISM

Drugs may be metabolized in many sites in the body, including the skin, gut, and lungs, but the liver is the primary location for drug metabolism. Many drugs are biotransformed in the liver to more water-soluble compounds before elimination from the body. These changes may occur as a result of phase I cytochrome P450 enzyme reactions, such as oxidation, reduction, and hydrolysis, or phase II conjugation reactions, such as glucuronidation, sulfation, or acetylation.[27]

Physiolgic Changes

Age-related physiologic changes in the liver include a reduction in size by 25% to 35%[28] and a decrease in hepatic blood flow of more than 40%.[22] Hepatocyte volume does not appear to change with age nor do liver function chemistries.[15,22] The rate of drug metabolism in the liver is determined by hepatic blood flow and enzyme activity in hepatocytes (intrinsic clearance).[9] The metabolism of drugs with high extraction ratios is limited by the rate of blood flow to the liver. Propranolol, calcium channel blockers, and tricyclic antidepressants are examples of such "flow-limited" drugs. Drugs such as warfarin and phenytoin have low intrinsic clearance and are slowly metabolized by hepatic enzymes.[24] These drugs are less prone to decreased or prolonged metabolism as a result of age-related alterations.[13]

Enzyme Changes

The metabolism of drugs via phase II reactions appears unchanged with aging, but there is still some question regarding age-related changes in phase I metabolism. The activity of cytochrome P450 enzymes has been studied in both in vitro and in vivo investigations and does not appear to change in old age. Studies of cytochrome P450 activity using the erythromycin breath test, in which exhaled carbon-14–tagged carbon dioxide is measured after intravenous injection with tagged erythromycin, have shown no age-related changes.[29] One study of human microsomal liver specimens showed no difference between older and younger patients in enzyme activity, including cytochrome P450 1A2, 2C, 2D6, and 3A, which are responsible for the metabolism of many drugs.[30,31]

Despite this finding, there appear to be age-dependent differences in metabolic clearance of many drugs, including benzodiazepines, theophylline, imipramine, propranolol, and indomethacin.[13] Alprazolam and diazepam are biotransformed by phase I enzymes to active metabolites, which may have a longer duration of action in elderly patients, whereas lorazepam and oxazepam undergo conjugation to inactive metabolites and are not affected by aging.[24] These decreases are more likely caused by reduced hepatic blood flow than specific alterations to liver enzymes. It is important to keep in mind that polypharmacy may have a significant effect on hepatic metabolism, because aside from being substrates for phase I enzymes, many drugs either inhibit or induce their activity.

EXCRETION

Drugs may be eliminated via the urine, feces, bile, or lungs. The route of particular interest in a discussion of age-related pharmacokinetic changes is renal excretion.

Table 4	
Selected medications that may require adjustment in renal dysfunction	
Pharmacologic Class	**Drug**
Antibiotics	Aminoglycosides
	Cephalosporins
	Fluoroquinolones
	Penicillins
Anticonvulsants	Gabapentin
	Oxcarbazepine
	Primidone
Cardiovascular agents	Lisinopril
	Ramipril
	Sotalol
	Diuretics
	Digoxin
Miscellaneous	Enoxaparin
	Morphine
	Metformin

The kidney decreases in size by 20% to 30% between 30 and 80 years of age, and microscopic analysis of the older kidney has shown increased fibrosis and tubular atrophy.[4] Reductions in renal function significantly affect the elimination of diuretics, digoxin, lithium, and other water-soluble drugs,[14] but much of this decline appears to be caused by morbidities commonly associated with age, rather than the natural aging process. A list of selected medication that may require adjustment in renal impairment may be found in **Table 4**.

Serum creatinine is widely used as a marker of renal function in clinical practice; however, creatinine alone is not an adequate measure of renal function in older patients. Elderly patients with decreased muscle mass may have serum creatinine levels within the normal range (usually 0.8 to 1.3 mg/dL) but in fact have significantly compromised renal function.[32] Therefore, calculating creatinine clearance, either from a urine collection or by using a mathematical equation such as the Cockcroft-Gault formula, is a more appropriate way to estimate kidney function.

Glomerular Filtration Rate

The glomerular filtration rate (GFR), an important marker of renal function, appears to be significantly affected by disease states such as hypertension, vascular disease, renal disease, heart failure, and malnutrition. Although cross-sectional studies have investigated the effect of age on renal function, the inclusion of patients with cormorbid conditions often confounds the effects of age.[33]

The question of whether GFR declines as a result of natural aging has been widely studied. The Baltimore Longitudinal Study of Aging found that one-third of normotensive elderly patients had no decline in GFR and that decreases in GFR correlated with increases in blood pressure. The authors concluded this decline was likely the result of microvascular disease, although they admitted it was impossible to determine whether renal disease or hypertension was the initial etiology.[34] Fliser and colleagues[35] then showed that GFR is only slightly lower in normotensive elderly individuals with normal dietary protein intake than in younger subjects and that renal function appears to be preserved until the eighth decade of life for healthy men and women. However, in clinical practice, the assumption of reduced kidney function with aging, whether as a result of disease progression or the natural aging process, influences the dosing strategies of medications excreted by the kidneys. A strategy of "start low, go slow" is a prudent one when prescribing renally eliminated drugs in elderly patients.

Effects of Declining Kidney Function on Drug Clearance

Mühlberg and Platt[36] performed pharmacokinetic studies in elderly patients, which have included angiotensin-converting enzyme inhibitors, nonsteroidal anti-inflammatory drugs, beta blockers, bronchodilators, diuretics, and benzodiazepines. These drugs include those eliminated primarily by glomerular filtration and tubular absorption as well as those metabolized by the liver. A creatinine clearance less than 40 mL/min was found to be associated with increased steady state concentrations of enalaprilat, cefotaxime, furosemide, spironolactone, hydrochlorothiazide, piracetam, pentoxifylline, and lorazepam, and dose reductions were recommended for these drugs. In another study, equivalent digoxin doses resulted in plasma concentrations that were almost twice as high in elderly patients as in younger patients, and digoxin clearance was found to be directly correlated to creatinine clearance. Lower initial doses of digoxin are recommended in elderly patients.[37]

PHARMACODYNAMICS

Pharmacodynamics is the study of the physiologic and biochemical effects that drugs have on the body. The magnitude of a drug's pharmacologic effect depends on the number and affinity of receptors at the site of action, signal transduction, and regulation of homeostasis.[13] Although there are several decades worth of clinical data available on pharmacokinetics in the elderly, there is much less concerning altered pharmacodynamics in this population. Studies have described increased sensitivity to cardiovascular medications, anticoagulants, benzodiazepines, and general anesthetics[14,17] that cannot be ascribed entirely to altered pharmacokinetics, but the mechanisms of action for these changes are, for the most part, still unclear. Proposed mechanisms of action include altered concentrations of neurotransmitters and receptors, hormonal changes, and impaired glucose metabolism.[9] Altered homeostatic mechanisms, such as impaired reflex tachycardia and impaired regulation of temperature and electrolytes, may also result in an increased risk for adverse drug effects.[38]

Cardiovascular System

The effects of calcium channel blockers are altered in elderly patients. In clinical studies, elderly hypertensive subjects experienced a greater decrease in systolic blood pressure in response to both diltiazem and verapamil than younger subjects, but whereas younger subjects experienced rebound tachycardia, this response was not seen in the elderly.[39,40] Diminished baroreceptor sensitivity, possibly mediated by reduced cardiac muscarinic receptor activity, may be partially responsible for these effects.[13,41]

The sensitivity of β-adrenoreceptors also appears to decline with age. In animal studies, an age-related decrease was seen in the tachycardia response to isoproterenol, a nonselective β-adrenoreceptor agonist. The authors concluded this likely was caused by diminished postreceptor activation of adenylate cyclase as opposed to reduced receptor number.[39] However, a study of β-adrenergic systems in the human heart found that β_1 receptor density and agonist affinity declined with age.[42] These changes in receptor activity may account for the reduced effectiveness of β-blockers compared with other antihypertensive agents in elderly patients.[43]

The effectiveness of loop diuretics, such as furosemide, is reduced in older patients. Decreases in kidney function result in reduced delivery of loop diuretics to their site of action in the nephron.[13] Heart failure patients in need of diuresis may require the addition of a diuretic for a different site of action in the kidney, such as the thiazidelike diuretic metaxalone.[44]

Respiratory System

Changes in the β-adrenergic system may also affect respiratory medications. Impaired postreceptor signaling may result in a decreased affinity at human lymphocyte receptor sites[39] and subsequent diminished response to β agonist bronchodilators. One study found that elderly patients experienced an attenuated response to the inhaled β_2 agonist albuterol after methacholine challenge.[45] However, a more recent investigation found no difference in response to albuterol between young and elderly subjects.[46]

Central Nervous System

Increased sensitivity to central nervous system–active medications in advanced age has been reported for benzodiazepines, antipsychotics, and antidepressants. Animal studies have found alterations in the disposition of dopamine, γ-aminobutyric-acid, and N-methyl-D-aspartate receptors in the brain.[13] Changes in the central noradrenergic, muscarinic, and serotonergic systems have also been reported. These alterations may lead to increased risk and magnitude of many common adverse effects including sedation, extrapyramidal symptoms, arrhythmias, confusion, insomnia, tremor, xerostomia and constipation.[47]

The pharmacodynamic response of the elderly to benzodiazepines has been well described. Sensitivity to diazepam increases 2-fold to 3-fold with aging, and these differences cannot be entirely attributed to increased blood concentrations.[48] Increased sedation and slower reaction time were seen in the elderly after administration of intravenous midazolam compared with younger subjects, even after accounting for differences in pharmacokinetic parameters.[49] Rissman and colleagues[50] postulated that altered composition and binding properties of benzodiazepine receptors may explain the enhanced pharmacologic response to benzodiazepines seen in elderly patients. Increased sensitivity to benzodiazepines is of considerable clinical importance because of the association between this class of drugs, falls, and hip fractures.[4]

Geriatric patients are more sensitive to the adverse effects of antipsychotic drugs than younger patients, particularly sedation, anticholinergic effects, orthostatic hypotension, and arrythmias.[14] Decreasing numbers of dopaminergic neurons and receptors, as well as diminished dopamine content in the brain, make elderly patients more susceptible to extrapyramidal effects of antipsychotics, especially akathisia, tardive dyskinesia, and psuedoparkinsonism.[13,51] Older individuals also have altered responses to opioid medications. Cepeda and coworkers[52] found that patients older than 60 years had a 2- to 8-fold higher risk of respiratory depression compared with younger patients, whereas the incidence of nausea and vomiting decreased. Central nervous system effects such as hallucinations and cognitive impairment may increase the risk of falls and subsequent fractures in older patients.[53]

IMPLICATIONS FOR POLYPHARMACY

Elderly patients are frequently prescribed complex drug regimens, by multiple prescribers, to treat conditions common in advanced age, such as coronary heart disease, heart failure, and diabetes. Often, each disease state is treated with several drugs that work synergistically to optimize outcomes.[38] Add to this the use of over-the-counter, herbal, or alternative medications, and the potential for unwanted effects, including decreased efficacy of prescription drugs or increased risk of side effects, is formidable. The altered action and disposition of drugs in the elderly patient should be taken into account by health care professionals to improve adherence, provide appropriate counseling, minimize side effects, and reduce medication errors.

ADVERSE DRUG REACTIONS

Adverse drug reactions are responsible for considerable morbidity and mortality in the elderly population and are a financial burden to the health care system. Adverse drug reactions in older adults are more likely to be severe and tend to be underreported.[4] At least 10% of hospital admissions for elderly patients may be caused by adverse drug reactions, and the mortality rate as a result of adverse drug reactions is significantly higher than that in younger patients.[54] Drugs taken to treat the same condition, for instance hypertension, predictably have synergistic effects that may lead to adverse effects such as dizziness and lightheadedness, increasing the risk for falls. Other commonly experienced adverse effects associated with polypharmacy in an elderly population are QT interval prolongation and hypoglycemia.

Prolongation of the QT interval

Elderly patients are more susceptible than younger patients to acquired prolongation of the QT interval, which may lead to arrhythmias, especially Torsades de Pointes and, subsequently, ventricular fibrillation. A study of QT intervals in healthy patients showed that elderly patients were more prone to prolonged QT intervals, which may be caused by cardiac hypertrophy, increased vascular stiffness, and other cardiac changes that occur with aging.[55] Patients over the age of 55 are at an increased risk for sudden cardiac death as a result of prolonged QT interval.[56] This risk may be further increased when multiple QT-prolonging drugs are added to a patient's regimen. Drugs from multiple pharmacologic classes may prolong the QT interval, including anti-infectives, antiarrhythmics, antidepressants, and antipsychotics.

Hypoglycemia

The treatment of type 2 diabetes mellitus is complicated in geriatric patients by a number of conditions, including impaired renal and cognitive function, comorbid disease states, and polypharmacy. Hypoglycemia may develop as a result of excess exogenous insulin or treatment with oral insulin secretagogues. The risk of hypoglycemia and its associated complications increases as the intensity of glycemic control increases. Older patients with an A_{1c} less than 7% are at an increased risk for falls,[57] and the elderly are more likely to need emergency treatment for hypoglycemic episodes.[58] Hypoglycemia is associated with more episodes of cardiac ischemia than are hyper- or normoglycemic states.[59] Severe episodes of hypoglycemia are associated with an increased risk for the development of dementia, especially in patients who have a history of multiple episodes.[60]

Sulfonylureas are the class of oral medications most likely to cause hypoglycemia in patients with diabetes, because they stimulate the release of insulin from functioning pancreatic beta cells.[6] First-generation sulfonylureas, such are chlorpropamide, are not recommended in older patients because of their long duration of action. The second-generation sulfonylureas glyburide and glimepiride each have at least 1 active metabolite that may accumulate in patients with impaired renal function and increase the risk of hypoglycemia. Glipizide, which has no active metabolites, may be a better choice in this population. Meglitinides, a nonsulfonylurea class of insulin secreta-gogues, also have the potential to cause hypoglycemia, but the risk is lower because of their shorter duration of action.[61] Metformin, commonly used as a first-line treatment in patients with type 2 diabetes, has little risk of hypoglycemia, but cannot be used in patients with significant renal impairment or uncompensated heart failure.

Patients with diabetes who are also taking β-blockers are at risk for hypoglycemia and masked symptoms of hypoglycemia. Epinephrine released as a result of hypoglycemia acts on β_1 receptors to increase heart rate and force of contraction, and β_2 receptors to increase glycogenolysis in the liver and glucagon release from the pancreas.

As with other medical conditions, many major clinical trials used to develop treatment guidelines have excluded older patients; however, the accepted glycemic target of A_{1c} less than 7% is considered acceptable for most elderly patients.[62] The American Geriatric Society suggests that for frail older adults or those with a life expectancy of 5 years, a less-stringent target may be appropriate.[63]

DRUG INTERACTIONS

Drug interactions are a particular problem in patients taking multiple medications. Drugs can interact with other drugs, herbal supplements, food, and disease states. Drugs interact when they have opposing effects, as occurs with nonsteroidal anti-inflammatory drugs and diuretics, or synergistic effects, as with sedation from benzodiazepines and anticholinergic drugs.[64] Many drugs affect the pharmacokinet-ics of other drugs, particularly those that are metabolized by the hepatic cytochrome P450 system.

Drugs may inhibit or induce the action of one or more hepatic enzymes (**Table 5**). Enzyme inhibitors increase the half-life of drugs that are enzyme substrates, whereas enzyme inducers decrease a substrate's half-life. Drugs with narrow therapeutic indices, such as warfarin, are more likely display clinically relevant pharmacodynamic alterations as a result of drug interactions.

Warfarin

Warfarin is an anticoagulant that exerts its activity by inhibiting the reduction of vitamin K in the liver, a process that is vital for the formation of clotting factors II, VII, IX, and X. It is used most commonly to prevent arterial thromboembolism in patients with atrial fibrillation or prosthetic heart valves. Although the risk for thromboembo-lism—and subsequent need for anticoagulation—increases with age, the risk for hemorrhage associated with anticoagulant therapy also increases, especially in the population of older adults with atrial fibrillation.[65] The effectiveness of warfarin is determined using the International Normalized Ratio (INR). Polypharmacy and drug interactions often are responsible for upsetting the delicate balance between antico-agulation and hemorrhage.

Warfarin is extensively metabolized by the cytochrome P450 enzymes 2C9, 2C19, 1A2, and 3A4.[59] Drugs that inhibit these enzymes can increase the INR, and potentially increase the risk for bleeding, whereas drugs that induce these enzymes may decrease the INR and consequently decrease the effectiveness of warfarin. Because the mechanism of action of warfarin involves the inhibition of vitamin K reductase, alterations in vitamin K intake may affect INR. Foods high in vitamin K include leafy greens, liver, and chick peas. Nutritional supplements and multivitamins are also sources of vitamin K.

Other mechanisms may also affect the action of warfarin. The risk of bleeding may be increased via pharmacodynamic interactions with antiplatelet drugs such as

Table 5
Selected medications and their interaction with the ctyochrome P450 system

	Substrates	Inhibitors	Inducers
CYP1A2	Amitriptyline Clozapine Diazepam Propranolol R-warfarin Theophylline	Cimetidine Erythromycin Isoniazid Ketoconazole	Cigarette smoke Phenobarbital Rifampin
CYP2C9	Celecoxib Fluoxetine Glipizide Losartan Phenytoin S-warfarin	Amiodarone Cimetidine Fluconazole Fluoxetine	Aprepitant Phenobarbital Rifampin
CYP2C19	Fluoxetine Methadone Phenobarbital Phenytoin R-warfarin	Clopidogrel Fluconazole Isoniazid Ketoconazole Omeprazole	Carbamazepine Phenytoin Rifampin St John's Wort
CYP2D6	Amitriptyline Carvedilol Fluoxetine Methadone Metoclopramide Oxycodone Promethazine	Amiodarone Bupropion Cimetidine Fluoxetine Paroxetine Quinidine Ritonavir	Rifampin
CYP3A4	Alprazolam Amiodarone Amlodipine Carbamazepine Fentanyl Haloperidol Losartan Methadone Mirtazapine R-warfarin Simvastatin Tramadol	Amiodarone Cimetidine Cyclosporine Diltiazem Erythromycin Fluconazole Fluoxetine Ketoconazole	Carbamazepine Dexamethasone Oxcarbazepine Phenobarbital Phenytoin Rifampin St John's Wort Topiramate

aspirin and clopidogrel. Patients taking nonsteroidal anti-inflammatory drugs while on oral anticoagulation therapy are at a higher risk for gastrointestinal bleeding, particularly those patients over the age of 60.[66] Warfarin is highly protein bound and has a narrow therapeutic index, which means that it may be displaced from albumin by other protein-bound drugs, increasing the free fraction of warfarin and potentially increasing the risk for bleeding.

SUMMARY

The population of older adults continues to increase, and polypharmacy in this population is more the rule than the exception. Physiologic changes that occur with aging result in multiple alterations to the pharmacokinetics and pharmacodynamics of drugs, which, in turn, increase the risk of adverse drug reactions. Consideration of initial dose adjustment, along with frequent medication reconciliation and analysis of the medication list, are keys to providing optimal pharmaceutical care for elderly patients.

REFERENCES

1. Qiuping G, Dillon CF, Burt VL. Prescription drug use continues to increase: U.S. prescription drug data for 2007 2008. NCHS data brief, no 42. Hyattsville (MD): National Center for Health Statistics; 2010. p. 7.
2. Patterns of medication use in the United States: A report from the Slone survey. Boston (MA): Slone Epidemiology Center at Boston University; 2006. p. 24.
3. Richter C. Oxidative damage to mitochondrial DNA and its relationship to ageing. Int J Biochem Cell Biol 1995;27(7):647–53.
4. McLean AJ, Le Couter DG. Aging biology and geriatric clinical pharmacology. Pharmacol Rev 2004;56:163–84.
5. Higami Y, Shimokawa I. Apoptosis in the aging process. Cell Tissue Res 2000;301: 125–32.
6. Le Couter DG, Hilmer SN, Glasgow N, et al. Prescribing in older people. Aust Fam Physician 2004; 33(10):777–81.
7. Cohen JS. Avoiding adverse reactions: Effective lower-dose drug therapies for older patients. Geriatrics. 2000; 55(2):54–64.
8. Wilkinson GR. The effects of diet, aging and disease-states on presystemic elimination and oral drug bioavailability in humans. Adv Drug Deliv Rev 1997; 129–59.
9. Corsonello A, Pedone C, Antonelli Incalzi R. Age-related pharmacokinetic and pharmacodynamic changes and related risk of adverse drug reactions. Curr Med Chem 2010;17:571–84.
10. Orr WC, Chen CL. Aging and neural control of the GI tract IV. Clinical and physiological aspects of gastrointestinal motility and aging. Am J Physiol Gastrointest Liver Physiol 2002;283:G1226–31.
11. Russell RM. Changes in gastrointestinal function attributed to aging. Am J Clin Nutr 1992;55:1203S–7S.
12. Schmucker DL. Aging and drug disposition: an update. Pharmacol Rev 1985; 37(2):133–46.
13. Turnheim K. Drug dosage in the elderly. Is it rational? Drugs Aging 1998;13(5):357–79.
14. Mangoni AA, Jackson SHD. Age-related changes in pharmacokinetics and pharmacodynamics: basic principles and practical applications. Br J Clin Pharmacol 2003; 1(57):6–14.
15. Eldesoky ES. Pharmacokinetic-pharmacodynamic crisis of the elderly. Am J Ther 2007;14:488–98.
16. Davies RO, Gomez HJ, Irwin JD, et al. An overview of the pharmacology of enalapril. Br J Clin Pharmacol 1984;18:215S–29S.
17. Shi S, Morike K, Klotz U. The clinical implications of ageing for rational drug therapy. Eur J Clin Pharmacol 2008;64:183–99.
18. Allen S. Are inhaled systemic therapies a viable option for the treatment of the elderly patient? Drugs Aging 2008;25(2):89–94.
19. Barrons R, Pegram A, Borries A. Inhaler device selection: Special considerations in elderly patients with chronic obstructive pulmonary disease. Am J Health-Syst Pharm 2011;68:1221–32.
20. Kaestli L, Wasilewski-Rasca A, Bonnabry P, et al. Use of transdermal drug formulations in the elderly. Drugs Aging 2008;25(4):269–80.

21. Starner CI, Gray SL, Guay D, et al. Geriatrics. In: DiPiro JT, Talbert RL, Yee GC, et al, editors. Pharmacotherapy: a pathophysiologic approach. 7th edition. New York: McGraw-Hill Medical; 2008. p. 57–66.
22. Schmucker DL. Liver function and phase I metabolism in the elderly: a paradox. Drugs Aging 2001;18(11):837–51.
23. Benet LZ, Hoener B. Changes in plasma protein binding have little clinical relevance. Clin PharmTher 2002;71(3):115–21.
24. Chutka DS, Evans JM, Fleming KC, et al. Drug prescribing for elderly patients. Mayo Clin Proc 1995;70(7):685–93.
25. Brenner SS, Klotz U. P-glycoprotein function in the elderly. Eur J Clin Pharmacol 2004;60:97–102.
26. Toornvliet R, van Berckel B, Luurtsema G, et al. Effect of age on functional P-glyco-protein in the blood-brain barrier measured by use of (R)-[(11C)verapamil and positron emission tomography. Clin Pharmacol Ther 2006;79:540–8.
27. Klotz U. Pharmacokinetics and drug metabolism in the elderly. Drug Met Rev 2009;41(2):67–76.
28. Le Couter DG, McLean AJ. The aging liver: drug clearance and oxygen diffusion barrier hypothesis. Clin Pharmacokinet 1998;34(5):359–73.
29. Watkins PB, Murray SA, Winkelman LG, et al. Erythromycin breath test as an assay of glucocorticoid-induced liver cytochromes P-450. J Clin Invest 1989;83:688–97.
30. Shimada T, Yamazaki H, Mimura M, et al. Interindividual variations in human liver cytochrome P-450 enzymes involved in the oxidation of drugs, carcinogens and toxic chemicals: studies with liver microsomes of 30 Japanese and 30 Caucasians. J Pharmacol Exp Ther 1994;270(1):414–21.
31. Delafuente, JC. Pharmacokinetic and pharmacodynamic alterations in the geriatric patient. Consult Pharm 2008; 23(4):324–34.
32. Swedko PJ. Serum creatinine is an inadequate screening test for renal failure in elderly patients. Arch Intern Med 2003;163:356–60.
33. Fliser D, Franek E, Ritz E. Renal function in the elderly—is the dogma of an inexorable decline of renal function correct? Nephrol Dial Transplant 1997;12:1553–5.
34. Lindeman RD, Tobin JD, Shock NW. Association between blood pressure and the rate of decline in renal function with age. Kidney Int 1984;26:861–8.
35. Fliser D, Zeier M, Nowack R, et al. Renal functional reserve in healthy elderly subjects. J Am Soc Nephrol 1993;3:1371–7.
36. Mülberg W, Platt D. Age-dependent changes of the kidneys: pharmacological impli-cations. Gerontology 1999;243–53.
37. Ewy GA, Kapadia GG, Yao L, et al. Digoxin metabolism in the elderly. Circulation 1969;39:449–53.
38. Jesson B. Minimising the risks of polypharmacy. Nurs Older People 2011;23(4):14–20.
39. Montamat SC, Abernethy DR. Calcium antagonists in geriatric patients: diltiazem in elderly persons with hypertension. Clin Pharmacol Ther 1989;45:682–91.
40. Abernethy DR, Schwartz JB, Todd EL, et al. Verapamil pharmacodynamics in young and elderly hypertensive patients: altered electrocardiographic and hypotensive re-sponses. Ann Intern Med 1986;105(3):329–36.
41. Docherty JR. Cardiovascular responses in ageing. Pharmacol Rev 1990;42(2):103–25.
42. White M, Roden R, Minobe W, et al. Age-related changes in β-adrenergic neuroef-fector systems in the human heart. Circulation 1994;3(90):1225–38.
43. Grossman E, Messerli FH. Why β-blockers are not cardioprotective in elderly patients with hypertension. Current Cardiol Rep 2002;4:468–73.
44. Aronow WS, Frishman WH, Cheng-Lai A. Cardiovascular drug therapy in the elderly. Cardiol Rev 2007;15(4):195–215.

45. Connolley MJ, Crowley JJ, Charan NB, et al. Impaired bronchodilator response to albuterol in healthy elderly men and women. Chest 1995;108:401–6.

46. Parker AL. Aging does not affect beta-agonist responsiveness after methacholine-induced bronchoconstriction. J Am Geriatr Soc 2004;52:388–92.

47. Lotrich FE, Pollock BG. Aging and clinical pharmacology: implications for antidepressants. J Clin Pharmacol 2005;45:1106–22.

48. Cook PT, Flanagan R, James IM. Diazepam tolerance: effect of age, regular sedation, and alcohol. BMJ 1984;289(6441):351–3.

49. Platten HP, Schweizer E, Dilger K, et al. Pharmacokinetics and pharmacodynamic action of midazolam in young and elderly patients undergoing tooth extraction. Clin Pharm Ther 1998;63(5):552–60.

50. Rissman RA, Nocera R, Fuller LM, et al. Age-related alterations in GABAA receptor subunits in the nonhuman primate hippocampus. Brain Res 2006;1073-1074:120–30.

51. Maxiner SM, Mellow AM, Tandon R. The efficacy, safety, and tolerability of antipsychotics in the elderly. J Clin Psychiatry 1999;60(Suppl 8):29–41.

52. Cepeda MS, Farrar JT, Baumgarten M, et al. Side effects of opioids during short-term administration: effects of age, gender, and race. Clin Pharm Ther 2003;74(2):102–12.

53. Pergolizzi J, Boger RH, Budd K, et al. Opioids and the management of chronic pain in the elderly: consensus statement of an international expert panel with focus on the six clinically most often used World Health Organization step III opioids (buprenorphine, fentanyl, hydromorphone, methadone, morphine, oxycodone). Pain Prac 2008;8(4):287–313.

54. Atkin PA, Veitch PC, Veitch EM, et al. The epidemiology of serious adverse drug reactions among the elderly. Drugs Aging 1999;14(2):141–52.

55. Mangoni AA, Kinirons MT, Swift CG, et al. Impact of age on QT interval and QT dispersion in healthy subjects: a regression analysis. Age Ageing 2003;32(3):326–31.

56. Straus S, Kors JA, De Bruin ML, et al. Prolonged QTc interval and risk of sudden cardiac death in a population of older adults. J Am Coll Cardiol 2006;47(2):362–7.

57. Nelson JM, Dufraux K, Cook PF. The relationship between glycemic control and falls in older adults. JAGS 2007;55:2041–4.

58. Leese GP, Wang J, Broomhill J, et al. Frequency of severe hypoglycemia requiring emergency treatment in type 1 and type 2 diabetes. Diabetes Care 26(4):1176–80.

59. Desouza C, Salazar H, Cheong B, et al. Association of hypoglycemia and cardiac ischemia: a study based on continuous monitoring. Diabetes Care 2003;26(5):1485–9.

60. Whitmer RA, Karter AJ, Yaffe K, et al. Hypoglycemic episodes and risk of dementia in older patients with type 2 diabetes mellitus. JAMA 2009;301(15):1565–72.

61. DRUGDEX® System. Thomson Reuters (Healthcare) Inc. Available at: http://www.thomsonhc.com. Accessed August 29, 2011.

62. Fravel MA, McDaniel DL, Ross MB, et al. Special considerations for treatment of type 2 diabetes mellitus in the elderly. Am J Health-Syst Pharm 2011;68:500–9.

63. Brown AF, Mangione CM, Saliba D, et al. California Healthcare Foundation/American Geriatrics Society Panel on Improving Care for Elders with Diabetes. Guidelines for improving the care of the older person with diabetes. J Am Geriatr Soc 2003;51(Suppl 5 Guidelines):S265–80.

64. Hobson M. Medications in older patients. West J Med 1992;157:539–43.

65. Torn M, Bollen W, van der Meer F, et al. Risks of oral anticoagulant therapy with increasing age. Arch Intern Med 2005;165:1527–32.

66. Lanza FL, Chan FK, Quigley EM, et al. Guidelines for prevention of NSAID-related ulcer complications. Am J Gastroenterol 2009;104:728–38.

Medication Adherence to Multidrug Regimens

Zachary A. Marcum, PharmD, MS[a], Walid F. Gellad, MD, MPH[b,c,d],*

KEYWORDS

- Medication • Adherence • Polypharmacy • Elderly
- Geriatric

Older adults are the largest consumers of medication in the United States, largely because of an age-associated increase in chronic conditions.[1] Because of this, multiple medication use (ie, polypharmacy) is a common consequence of providing health care to older adults.[2] Polypharmacy is of particular concern to older adults because they may have unique barriers and challenges to managing multidrug regimens, including cognitive impairment, functional limitations, financial restraints, use of multiple health care providers, or transportation limitations, to name a few.[2,3] In addition, one of the most significant potential consequences of polypharmacy could be its impact on medication adherence in the older adult.

Medication adherence can be defined as "the extent to which a person's behavior (in this case, taking medication) corresponds with agreed recommendations from a health care provider."[4] Widely varying rates of nonadherence have been reported previously depending on the definition of nonadherence, the population studied, and the length of observation; yet, multiple reviews on medication adherence report that approximately 50% of older adults do not adhere to at least one of their chronic medications.[4,5] Moreover, it is important to identify the specific type of nonadherence within the medication use process—nonfulfillment (or primary nonadherence), nonpersistence, or nonconforming.[6] Primary nonadherence occurs when the provider

Dr Marcum is supported by a National Institute on Aging grant (P30AG024827), and Dr Gellad is supported by a VA Career Development Award (09-207).

Disclosure: Dr Gellad has received an honorarium from Vindico Medical Education for preparation of a continuing medical education (CME) activity focused on improving medication adherence.

[a] Department of Medicine (Geriatrics), School of Medicine, University of Pittsburgh, 3471 Fifth Avenue, Suite 500, Pittsburgh, PA 15213, USA

[b] Center for Health Equity Research and Promotion, VA Pittsburgh Healthcare System, 7180 Highland Drive, Pittsburgh, PA 15206, USA

[c] Department of Medicine (General Medicine), School of Medicine, University of Pittsburgh, Pittsburgh, 3471 Fifth Avenue, Suite 500, Pittsburgh, PA 15213, USA

[d] RAND Health, 4570 Fifth Avenue, Suite 600, Pittsburgh, PA 15213, USA

* Corresponding author. Center for Health Equity Research and Promotion, VA Pittsburgh Healthcare System, 7180 Highland Drive, Pittsburgh, PA 15206.

E-mail address: Walid.gellad@va.gov

prescribes a medication, but it is never filled by the patient. Nonpersistence is when the patient decides to stop taking a medication after starting it, without being advised by a health professional to do so. Furthermore, so-called "nonconforming" nonadherence includes a variety of ways in which medications are not taken as prescribed (eg, taking incorrect doses, skipping doses, or taking doses at incorrect times).[3]

Thus, it is clear that taking medication is a complex behavior that requires multiple successful steps on the part of patients (ie, to fill, initiate, continue, and take the prescription as intended). Prescribers play important roles in the process as well, because they are ultimately responsible for prescribing the most appropriate medication and, along with other health care professionals, monitoring their use. Taken together, polypharmacy and medication adherence present a unique challenge for the older adult, their caregiver(s), and the health care team. In this review, we first discuss the various ways in which medication adherence is measured, and then we present a conceptual model, illustrating the complex interplay between polypharmacy and medication (non)adherence in older adults, summarize key literature on the topic, highlight strategies for improvement, and conclude by describing areas of uncertainty and priorities for future research.

MEASUREMENT

One of the greatest challenges in the field of adherence research is the accurate measurement of this complex health behavior. Various methods have been described, including using self-reported surveys, pill counts, drug levels, physiologic measures (eg, heart rate with β-blockers), pharmaceutical claims, electronic medication monitoring, and physician ordering in electronic health records. Each method has inherent limitations, and various iterations of each method have been used in previous studies, leading to substantial heterogeneity in the current evidence base.

It is commonly accepted that there is no "gold standard" for measuring medication adherence. However, because medication adherence is a complex health behavior, it may be more prudent to focus on which specific aspects of medication adherence each measure is actually capturing. For example, pharmaceutical claims have been used frequently in recent years to study medication adherence across multiple conditions using large insurance-based data sources by evaluating medication refill patterns.[7] This approach typically reports a proportion of days covered, a medication possession ratio (MPR), or a cumulative medication gap. That is, claims-based adherence studies are simply reporting on the rate of medication possession among patients and not the actual medication-taking itself. Moreover, these methods rely on at least 2 medication refills to be calculated, thus missing altogether the patient exhibiting primary nonadherence or nonpersistence after one refill.[8] Of note, electronic health records that track physician ordering and patient refilling of chronic medications also offer an opportunity to capture these important and often undocumented cases of primary nonadherence or nonpersistence.

Self-report is another common method used to measure medication adherence in older adults. Several self-reported measures have been published (**Fig. 1**), including the Morisky Medication Adherence Scales (a 4-item and a newer 8-item measure), various cost-related measures, and the Adherence Estimator.[9–12] The Adherence Estimator is a new 3-item measure that can be used to predict medication adherence in patients newly initiated on a chronic medication.[11] Self-reported measures offer the convenience of low respondent burden and minimal cost; however, there is the potential for social desirability bias (ie, patients may report what they think the clinician wants to hear and not their true medication-taking behavior). If prefaced

Morisky Medication Adherence Scale (4-item)*	Morisky Medication Adherence Scale (8-item)*	Adherence Estimator*
1. Do you ever forget to take your (name of health condition) medicine? 2. Do you ever have problems remembering to take your (name of health condition) medication?† 3. When you feel better, do you sometimes stop taking your (name of health condition) medicine? 4. Sometimes if you feel worse when you take your (name of health condition) medicine, do you stop taking it? *Morisky DE et al. Med Care 1986;24:67-74. †Modified from the original 1986 version	1. Do you sometimes forget to take your (health concern) pills? 2. People sometimes miss taking their medications for reasons other than forgetting. Thinking over the past two weeks, were there any days when you did not take your (health concern) medicine? 3. Have you ever cut back or stopped taking your medication without telling your doctor, because you felt worse when you took it? 4. When you travel or leave home, do you sometimes forget to bring along your (health concern) medication? 5. Did you take your (health concern) medicine yesterday? 6. When you feel like your (health concern) is under control, do you sometimes stop taking your medicine? 7. Taking medication every day is a real inconvenience for some people. Do you ever feel hassled about sticking to your (health concern) treatment plan? 8. How often do you have difficulty remembering to take all of your medications? *Morisky DE et al. J Clin Hypertens (Greenwich) 2008;10:348-54.	1. I am convinced of the importance of my prescription medication. 2. I worry that my prescription medication will do more harm than good to me. 3. I feel financially burdened by my out-of-pocket expenses for my prescription medication. *McHorney CA. Curr Med Res Opin 2009;25:215-38.

Fig. 1. Examples of self-reported medication adherence measures. *Data from* Refs[9–11]

appropriately in a nonaccusatory manner, self-reported measures can help understand the reasons for nonadherence, which may better identify areas for immediate intervention compared with impersonal measures such as pharmacy claims.

Finally, pill counts or electronic medication monitoring (eg, medication event monitoring system [MEMS]) are common approaches used in clinical trials to provide objective and quantitative measures of medication adherence. MEMS devices are limited by their high cost, restricting their widespread use. Moreover, pill counts provide an estimate of medication adherence based on the number of pills in the vial (usually for a single medication) but do not ensure that the patient actually took the medication (eg, in the case of a patient "pill dumping" before an appointment).

When comparing the psychometric properties across the various methods for measurement of adherence, large amounts of heterogeneity are present in the literature. Grymonpre and colleagues[13] compared medication adherence calculated using pill count, self-report, and pharmacy claims data in a sample of community-dwelling older adults (≥65 years) and found that the pill count method underestimated medication adherence. A recent meta-analysis examining the correlation between MEMS and self-reported questionnaires reported that these 2 measurements tend to be at least moderately correlated.[14] However, others have described the limitations of self-reported measures of medication adherence and called for attention to improving the development of such measures in future research.[15] While recognizing the inherent limitations for each method, the most robust approach may be to use multiple measurements to capture a broader range of adherence information in older adults.

Each of the methods described above is commonly used in adherence research, but simple measures of adherence for use in the clinical setting are difficult to come

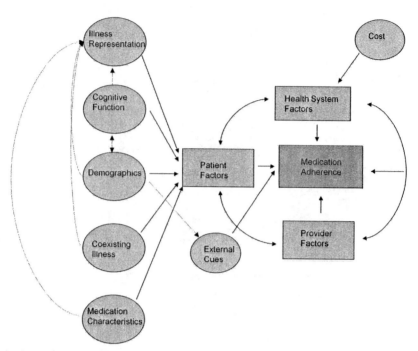

Fig. 2. General conceptual model of medication adherence and the interaction between patient factors. (*Adapted from* Gellad WF, Grenard J, McGlynn EA. A review of barriers to medication adherence: a framwork for driving policy options. RAND Corporation, 2009. http://www.rand.org/pubs/technical_reports/TR765. Reprinted with permission.)

by. Some clinical practices (as well as insurers and pharmacy benefit managers) have begun to provide claims-based measures of adherence to the clinician in an effort to identify nonadherent patients at the time of the visit. Others may be using some of the self-reported measures in their clinic, although we are not aware of many examples of this approach currently in the literature. At the very least, all providers should be asking patients simple questions about any problems they may be having with their medications at each clinic visit.

CONCEPTUAL FRAMEWORK OF BARRIERS TO MEDICATION ADHERENCE

Extensive literature has been published on barriers to medication adherence in older adults.[3,5,6,16] In turn, various conceptual models have been proposed to illustrate the complex relationship in older adults between patient, health-system, and provider factors and medication adherence.[3,17,18] Yet, there is an apparent mismatch between these conceptual frameworks and the existing body of literature; for example, limited evidence is available assessing how the different barriers interact. Of importance to this review, polypharmacy is frequently studied as a potential barrier in adherence research, but it is unclear how polypharmacy affects (or is affected by) other barriers to either increase or decrease adherence.

For the current review, we adapted a conceptual framework for medication adherence in older adults proposed by Gellad and colleagues[3] (**Fig. 2**) originally modeled from the framework proposed by Park and Jones.[17] In the previous models, the complex interplay among patient, health-system, and provider factors are central

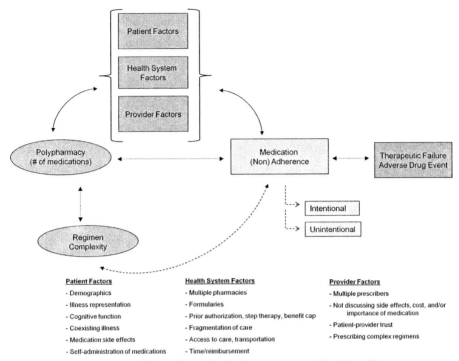

Fig. 3. Conceptual model of the effect of polypharmacy on medication adherence.

to their explanatory value. Not only do those factors interact, but each individual patient-level factor also interacts with other patient factors. For example, the presence of multiple comorbid conditions in a patient could affect the patient's perceived need for certain medications—in this case, comorbid conditions and perceived need for medications each affect adherence individually, but the interaction between the 2 may also affect adherence. In another example, cognitive function, another patient-level barrier to adherence, could affect the socioeconomic status of a patient (which, in turn, may be related to adherence), and it could also affect how patients perceive their need for medications.

Our proposed model focuses on the potential pathways from one of the medication characteristics in the previous model, polypharmacy, to medication (non)adherence, potentially being mediated by various patient, health-system or provider factors (**Fig. 3**). Polypharmacy can lead to medication nonadherence simply because of the greater number of medications that can be missed on a daily basis, yet polypharmacy can also lead to nonadherence through other mechanisms. Polypharmacy here is defined as the number of different medications a patient is prescribed and taking; this is distinct from the concept of regimen complexity, which encompasses the number of daily doses for a medication, the presence of nonoral routes of administration, and the need for specific dosing instructions (eg, warfarin, bisphosphonates). Regimen complexity is closely correlated with polypharmacy and has previously been found to be associated with lower medication adherence.[19] An additional important distinction highlighted in the model is the differentiation between intentional and unintentional medication nonadherence, which are 2 very different medication-taking behaviors. Distal health outcomes, including therapeutic failures and adverse drug events, are also included because they are significant consequences or causes of medication nonadherence.[20]

The following paragraphs on patient, health-system, and provider factors highlight potential mediators of the association between polypharmacy and medication nonadherence. These factors should not be considered in isolation; rather, they should be viewed as interacting with many other factors, and clinicians must evaluate each patient individually to assess their unique barriers as they change over time.

Patient Factors

Older adults may be influenced by various factors that could affect their medication-taking behavior, including demographic factors, such as socioeconomic status and age, cognitive function, coexisting illness, illness representation, and medication side effects, to name a few. Although these patient factors can affect medication adherence on their own, they can also both cause polypharmacy (eg, coexisting illnesses leading to more medications prescribed) and mediate the relationship between polypharmacy and nonadherence (eg, drug interactions and side effects are more likely when taking more medications). Patients' representations of their own illnesses can potentially be affected by their pill burden, and that representation has previously been shown to affect adherence.[17] In some cases, the beliefs that patients have about the number of medications they are taking, rather than the actual number, may have a stronger association with their adherence. For example, in a study of women taking osteoporosis medications, agreeing with the statement that one was taking too many different medications was a more important predictor of very low adherence (medication possession ratio <20%) than the actual number of medications taken.[21]

Health-System Factors

The most common health-system barrier to medication adherence is cost.[12,22] Cost is clearly more of a problem for those patients taking more medications, and thus polypharmacy may affect adherence through higher cost sharing. In addition, polypharmacy could lead to filling at multiple pharmacies depending on the type of medication, the type of providers, and the patient's insurance; older adults filling prescriptions at multiple pharmacies may face greater burden to adhering than those using a single pharmacy.[23] Moreover, formulary substitutions, prior authorization, fragmentation of care, and ability to access care are all potential barriers to medication adherence for the older adult and are likely to be even more significant in those taking multiple medications.

Provider Factors

Providers may unknowingly contribute to medication nonadherence by not discussing potential medication side effects or the importance of the medication or simply by prescribing complex regimens (when more simplified options are available). Patients receiving specialized care are often required to visit multiple providers and subsequently encounter multiple prescribers who may not be in communication with each other, thus, leading to unintended polypharmacy.

Although we make note of the above barriers, the list is by no means completely inclusive. Perhaps the most important concept when it comes to identifying barriers to medication adherence and how polypharmacy may lead to problems with adherence is that each patient will be different, for each medication they take, and at different points in time. Simply put, understanding the potential barriers patients face does nothing more than prepare clinicians to better understand what the specific patient in front of them might be facing.

EVIDENCE

Having discussed the conceptual framework for understanding how polypharmacy may be associated with medication adherence, we now discuss the current available evidence on the topic. Numerous reviews have been published on medication adherence in older adults, and polypharmacy has been one of the most commonly studied risk factors for nonadherence. Balkrishnan[16] conducted a review from 1962 to 1997 examining predictors of medication adherence in the elderly and found mixed results for the association between the number of medications and adherence. We recently conducted a systematic review from 1998 to 2010 focusing on older adults in the United States and, similarly, found mixed results for the association between polypharmacy and medication adherence.[6] This heterogeneity in the literature is consistent with other systematic reviews reporting on the relationship between polypharmacy and medication adherence.[24]

To build on the above reviews, we searched PubMed (through July 2011) and the reference lists of articles included in our prior review and found only 3 additional studies focusing on older adults examining polypharmacy and adherence. Thus, in total, we identified 9 articles for the purpose of this review (**Table 1**).[23,25–32] Among these 9 articles, 6 reported a negative association between greater number of medications and medication adherence, that is, the presence of more medications was associated with worse adherence. Alternatively, 1 study reported a positive association between polypharmacy and medication adherence, and 2 studies found no significant association. Importantly, when only assessing those studies using a more rigorous design (ie, excluding cross-sectional studies), 4 out of 5 studies reported that polypharmacy was associated with greater risk of nonadherence.

It is important to highlight that polypharmacy is often assessed along with multiple other covariates to determine their association with medication adherence in epidemiologic studies or during secondary analyses of previously completed trials. In other words, polypharmacy is rarely prespecified as the primary independent variable for predicting medication adherence, making it difficult to determine the true association between polypharmacy and medication adherence.

Taken together, there appears to be an association between polypharmacy and poorer medication adherence. However, it is difficult to be certain from the literature because of the mixed results, the likely unmeasured confounding, limited study designs (eg, cross sectional), small sample sizes, and limited generalizability. In addition, this uncertainty is surely a result of the complexity of measuring adherence—the interaction between polypharmacy and all the additional factors described above is impossible to capture in most studies, and the fact that adherence can vary for different medications within the same person at different times makes adherence an even more complicated behavior to quantify. Although the effect of polypharmacy on medication adherence may not be completely clear in the literature, improving medication adherence to maximize the therapeutic benefit of pharmacotherapy remains a cornerstone of geriatric care. We discuss some strategies for improving adherence below.

STRATEGIES FOR IMPROVING ADHERENCE

Several interventions have been trialed to find effective solutions for this ongoing public health problem in older adults, with minimal success to date.[5,33,34] In general,

Table 1
Studies reporting on the association between polypharmacy and medication adherence in older adults in the United States, 1998–2011

Citation	Study Design	Sample Description	Measure of Adherence	Polypharmacy Definition	Key Polypharmacy Findings
Chapman et al[25] (2008)	Observational cohort	Adults aged ≥65 years who initiated treatment with both AH and LL therapy within a 90-day period	Medication possession ratio (cutoff 80%)	No. of prescription medications	Adherence rate was decreased with taking more medications (AOR 0.43 for ≥6 medications vs 0–1 medication; 95% CI 0.36 to 0.50; $P<.001$).
Choudhry et al[23] (2011)	Observational cohort	Patients prescribed a statin or an ACE-inhibitor (mean age 63 years) (2 separate cohorts) from a large pharmacy benefit manager	Proportion of days covered (also assessed therapeutic complexity)	No. of prescription medications	Adherence was decreased with a greater number of medications in both cohorts (statin users: adjusted % change in adherence per additional medication, 0.89, $P<.001$; ACE-inhibitor users: adjusted % change in adherence per additional medication, 0.69, $P<.001$).
Gazmararian et al[26] (2006)	Observational cohort	Adults aged ≥65 years with coronary heart disease, diabetes, hyperlipidemia, or HTN	Cumulative medication gap <20%	No. of oral prescription medications (≤3 vs >3)	Multivariate analysis showed that those who took more medications had a lower odds of having nonadherence compared with those taking less medication (AOR 0.77; 95%, CI 0.73 to 0.95) after controlling for health literacy, age, race, sex, and education.
Grant et al[27] (2003)	Cross-sectional	Patients with diabetes (mean age 66 years) receiving primary care	Self-reported diabetes-related medication adherence	No. of prescription medications	Adherence was not significantly associated with the number of diabetes-related medications.

Source	Study design	Population	Adherence measure	Factor examined	Findings
Gray et al[28] (2001)	Observational cohort	Adults aged ≥65 years receiving home health care following hospitalization for medical illness	Underadherence: at least 1 medication <70%; Overadherence: at least one medication >120%	No. of prescription medications; Taking a drug ≥3 times/day	Multivariable analysis showed that *underadherence* was significantly associated with greater medication use (AOR 1.16, 95% CI 1.03 to 1.31) after controlling for demographic, health-related and medication-related covariates.
Ownby et al[29] (2006)	Cross-sectional	Patients with memory disorders cared for at a memory disorders clinic	Caregivers' reports of patients' medication adherence	No. of prescription medications	Adherence was not found to be associated with the number of medications.
Turner et al[30] (2009)	Cross-sectional	Adults aged ≥70 years with HTN	Self-reported not missing any medication in the past 3 months	Antihypertensive regimen complexity (≥4 medications)	Adherence was significantly negatively associated (less likely) with having ≥4 antihypertensive medications in regimen (AOR 0.23; 95% CI, 0.08 to 0.72).
Stoehr et al[31] (2008)	Cross-sectional	Adults aged ≥65 years cared for in 7 private office practices	Global judgment by research nurses (ie, dichotomous outcome, yes/no) after a home visit	No. of prescription medications (≥5 vs <5); Dosing frequency (≥4 vs <4 times/d)	Adherence was negatively associated with a greater number of prescription medications (OR 0.45; 95% CI, 0.21 to 0.95; $P = .04$).
van Bruggen et al[32] (2009)	Cluster-RCT	Patients with diabetes (mean age ~67 years) receiving primary care (Netherlands)	Medication possession ratio (cutoff 80%)	No. of prescription medications	Adherence to blood pressure lowering drugs was negatively associated with a greater number of prescription medications (AOR 0.84; 95% CI 0.78-91; $P<.0001$); however, adherence was not significantly associated with the number of oral blood glucose or cholesterol-lowering drugs.

Abbreviations: ACE, angiotensin-converting enzyme; AH, antihypertensive; AOR, adjusted odds ratio; CI, confidence interval; HTN, hypertension; LL, lipid lowering.

multifaceted interventions have been shown to have the most impact in elders (who are often receiving polypharmacy) to enhance medication adherence, making it difficult to disentangle the effective from the ineffective components.[5] There is evidence from clinical trials of the effectiveness of decreasing regimen complexity in improving adherence,[33] and some evidence from well-conducted natural experiments of lowering cost sharing to increase adherence (although these are not specific to older patients).[35] There is also evidence that pharmacist interventions can improve medication adherence and related health care utilization; yet, the effect of these interventions commonly dissipates upon discontinuation and their cost effectiveness is unclear.[36,37]

So what can we do to improve medication adherence in older adults in light of limited evidence available? The following are some key strategies that are rooted in the literature[2,38–40]:

1. **Promote rational, conservative prescribing—a necessary but not sufficient step alone.**[38] One of the most important strategies for improving adherence is to first make sure patients are receiving the most appropriate medications. Evaluate the medication regimen to ensure that it is appropriate, including discontinuing or dose adjusting any unnecessary medications or doses, decreasing regimen complexity, and minimizing cost sharing. Begin new medications only after assuring oneself and the patient and caregiver that the benefits outweigh the risks.
2. **Avoid the "prescribing cascade."**[40] If a patient has new symptoms after starting a medication (eg, pedal edema after starting a calcium channel blocker), try changing the medication before adding another one to treat the symptoms.
3. **Incorporate the measurement of medication adherence and individual-level risk factors for nonadherence into clinical practice.** With the uptake of health information technology, detecting medication adherence problems (at least problems with refilling medications or experiencing adverse drug events) may be more easily incorporated into the clinical encounter. Other screening tests may be available to detect different aspects of medication adherence (eg, taking medications incorrectly). Always solicit information from the patient/caregiver and incorporate a multidisciplinary approach when possible (using nurses and pharmacists) to monitor medication adherence over time.
4. **Evaluate for potential barriers in the older adult.** Knowing some of the more common barriers to adherence in older adults, ask about them during the clinical encounter, including (but not limited to): financial restraints (cost sharing), use of multiple pharmacies or prescribers, complex medication regimens, cognitive impairment, dexterity limitations, swallowing difficulty, and hearing or visual impairment.
5. **Take into account the patients' and caregivers' underlying beliefs about medication use.** Attention should be given to understanding patient beliefs about the necessity of the medications. Only then can patient-specific medication adherence recommendations be made and medication regimen monitoring plans developed and implemented.

LESSONS FOR FUTURE RESEARCH

Moving forward, there are clear gaps in the literature that deserve attention because of the considerable impact of medication nonadherence in a rapidly aging population. Based on an evaluation of published research and our own clinical experience, we offer some suggestions for future work to advance the study of medication adherence in older adults. First, the most evident cause of the heterogeneity in the literature is the lack of standardization of the measurement of medication adherence across studies, preventing pooling of results to better describe the effectiveness of interventions. Although we acknowledge that no one measure can capture the entire universe of medication adherence behavior, consistent use of reliable and valid instruments across studies and over time in large cohorts of older adults would allow for more systematic results and implications. Many researchers are now using the standard definitions of adherence and persistence as outlined by Cramer and coworkers.[41] Along those lines, there is a great need to study cohorts of older adults' medication-taking behavior over time to study all aspects of medication nonadherence within the same population (ie, primary nonadherence, nonpersistence, and nonconforming).

Second, future studies should report on any differential impact of interventions on intentional versus unintentional medication nonadherence. Interventions found to be effective for unintentional nonadherence (eg, using electronic reminder devices) will likely not be appropriate for older adults showing intentional nonadherence who may have knowingly stopped a medication. Such patients may benefit from an intervention that allows for a timely line of communication with a health care professional to address their key barrier(s).

Third, researchers should take seriously the call to develop larger, more rigorous, clinical trials testing interventions to improve adherence as well as distal outcomes (eg, adverse drug events and therapeutic failures).[5] The Institute of Medicine included interventions to improve adherence as one of the top 100 priorities for comparative effectiveness research.[42] Importantly, cost-effectiveness studies should be incorporated into studies of adherence interventions to make coherent policy arguments. Comparative effectiveness studies are needed comparing interventions of different lengths of time, and of different "intensities" (eg, single-faceted vs multifaceted interventions).

Finally, before attempting to improve medication adherence, it is critical to ensure that the medication regimen is the most appropriate one for the individual patient. Future trials could assess a stepwise approach to enhancing medication use by first determining any changes to improve medication appropriateness. Only after this has been done should interventions to improve medication adherence be trialed and implemented to avoid adherence to a suboptimal regimen. One intervention that will completely prevent nonadherence and limit polypharmacy is to stop a medication that is no longer clinically indicated or consistent with the patient's goals of care.[43]

SUMMARY

Despite the fact that medication adherence has been extensively described in the literature over the last several decades, a quote by Becker and Maiman from over 35 years ago best captures the current state of our understanding: "Patient compliance [sic adherence] has become the best documented, but least understood, health behavior."[44] Future research is greatly needed to identify and translate safe and effective interventions into routine clinical practice to improve adherence. Only then can we begin to make significant improvements to the medication use process and, in turn, the health of older adults.

ACKNOWLEDGMENTS

The authors thank Joseph T. Hanlon, PharmD, MS for reviewing an earlier draft of this manuscript.

REFERENCES

1. Qato DM, Alexander GC, Conti RM, et al. Use of prescription and over-the-counter medications and dietary supplements among older adults in the United States. JAMA 2008;300:2867–78.
2. Hajjar ER, Cafiero AC, Hanlon JT. Polypharmacy in elderly patients. Am J Geriatr Pharmacother 2007;5:345–51.
3. Gellad WF, Grenard J, McGlynn EA. A review of barriers to medication adherence: a framework for driving policy options. Santa Monica (CA): RAND Corporation, 2009.
4. Sabaté E. Adherence to long-term therapies: evidence for action. Geneva (Switzerland): World Health Organization (WHO); 2003.
5. Haynes RB, Ackloo E, Sahota N, et al. Interventions for enhancing medication adherence. Cochrane Database Syst Rev 2008;2:CD000011.
6. Gellad WF, Grenard JL, Marcum ZA. A systematic review of barriers to medication adherence in the elderly: looking beyond cost and regimen complexity. Am J Geriatr Pharmacother 2011;9:11–23.
7. Andrade SE, Kahler KH, Frech F, et al. Methods for evaluation of medication adherence and persistence using automated databases. Pharmacoepidemiol Drug Saf 2006; 15:565–74.
8. Raebel MA, Carroll NM, Ellis JL, et al. Importance of including early nonadherence in estimations of medication adherence. Ann Pharmacother 2011;45:1053–60.
9. Morisky DE, Green LW, Levine DM. Concurrent and predictive validity of a self-reported measure of medication adherence. Med Care 1986;24:67–74.
10. Morisky DE, Ang A, Kroussel-Wood M, et al. Predictive validity of a medication adherence measure in an outpatient setting. J Clin Hypertens (Greenwich) 2008;10:348–54.
11. McHorney CA. The Adherence Estimator: a brief, proximal screener for patient propensity to adhere to prescription medications for chronic disease. Curr Med Res Opin 2009;25:215–38.
12. Soumerai SB, Pierre-Jacques M, Zhang F, et al. Cost-related medication nonadherence among elderly and disabled Medicare beneficiaries: a national survey 1 year before the Medicare drug benefit. Arch Intern Med 2006;166:1829–35.
13. Grymonpre RE, Didur CD, Montgomery PR, et al. Pill count, self-report, and pharmacy claims data to measure medication adherence in the elderly. Ann Pharmacother 1998;32:749–54.
14. Shi L, Liu J, Fonesca V, et al. Correlation between adherence rates measured by MEMS and self-reported questionnaires: a meta-analysis. Health Qual Life Outcomes 2010;8:99.
15. Voils CI, Hoyle RH, Thorpe CT, et al. Improving the measurement of self-reported medication nonadherence. J Clin Epidemiol 2011;64:250–4.
16. Balkrishnan R. Predictors of medication adherence in the elderly. Clin Ther 1998;20:764–71.
17. Park DC, Jones TR. Medication adherence and aging. In: Fisk AD, Rogers WA, editors. Handbook of human factors and the older adult. San Diego (CA): Academic Press, Inc; 1997. p. 257–87.
18. Krousel-Wood M, Thomas S, Muntner P, et al. Medication adherence: a key factor in achieving blood pressure control and good clinical outcomes in hypertensive patients. Curr Opin Cardiol 2004;19:357–62.
19. Claxton AJ, Cramer J, Pierce C. A systematic review of the associations between dose regimens and medication compliance. Clin Ther 2001;23:1296–310.

20. Kaiser RM, Schmader KE, Pieper CF, et al. Therapeutic failure-related hospitalisations in the frail elderly. Drugs Aging 2006;23:579–86.

21. Solomon DH, Brookhart MA, Tsao P, et al. Predictors of very low adherence with medications for osteoporosis: towards development of a clinical prediction rule. Osteoporosis Int 2011;22:1737–43.

22. Madden JM, Graves AJ, Zhang F, et al. Cost-related medication nonadherence and spending on basic needs following implementation of Medicare Part D. JAMA 2008;299:1922–8.

23. Choudhry NK, Fischer MA, Avorn J, et al. The implications of therapeutic complexity on adherence to cardiovascular medications. Arch Intern Med 2011;171:814–22.

24. Vik SA, Maxwell CJ, Hogan DB. Measurement, correlates, and health outcomes of medication adherence among seniors. Ann Pharmacother 2004;38:303–12.

25. Chapman RH, Petrilla AA, Benner JS, et al. Predictors of adherence to concomitant antihypertensive and lipid-lowering medications in older adults: a retrospective, cohort study. Drugs Aging 2008;25:885–92.

26. Gazmararian JA, Kripalani S, Miller MJ, et al. Factors associated with medication refill adherence in cardiovascular-related diseases: a focus on health literacy. J Gen Intern Med 2006;21:1215–21.

27. Grant RW, Devita NG, Singer DE, et al. Polypharmacy and medication adherence in patients with type 2 diabetes. Diabetes Care 2003;26:1408–12.

28. Gray SL, Mahoney JE, Blough DK. Medication adherence in elderly patients receiving home health services following hospital discharge. Ann Pharmacother 2001;35:539–45.

29. Ownby RL, Hertzog C, Crocco E, et al. Factors related to medication adherence in memory disorder clinic patients. Aging Ment Health 2006;10:378–85.

30. Turner BJ, Hollenbeak C, Weiner MG, et al. Barriers to adherence and hypertension control in a racially diverse representative sample of elderly primary care patients. Pharmacoepidemiol Drug Saf 2009;18:672–81.

31. Stoehr GP, Lu SY, Lavery L, et al. Factors associated with adherence to medication regimens in older primary care patients: the Steel Valley Seniors Survey. Am J Geriatr Pharmacother 2008;6:255–63.

32. van Bruggen R, Gorter K, Stolk RP, et al. Refill adherence and polypharmacy among patients with type 2 diabetes in general practice. Pharmacoepidemiol Drug Saf 2009;18:983–91.

33. Kripalani S, Yao X, Haynes RB. Interventions to enhance medication adherence in chronic medical conditions: a systematic review. Arch Intern Med 2007;167:540–50.

34. Mahtani KR, Heneghan CJ, Glasziou PP, et al. Reminder packaging for improving adherence to self-administered long-term medications. Cochrane Databse Syst Rev 2011;9:CD005025.

35. Maciejewski ML, Farley JF, Parker J, et al. Copayment reductions generate greater medication adherence in targeted patients. Health Aff (Millwood) 2010;29:2002–8.

36. Lee JK, Grace KA, Taylor AJ. Effect of a pharmacy care program on medication adherence and persistence, blood pressure, and low-density lipoprotein cholesterol: a randomized controlled trial. JAMA 2006;296:2563–71.

37. Murray MD, Young J, Hoke S, et al. Pharmacist intervention to improve medication adherence in heart failure: a randomized trial. Ann Intern Med 2007;146:714–25.

38. Schiff GD, Galanter WL, Duhig J, et al. Principles of conservative prescribing. Arch Intern Med 2011;171:1433–40.

39. Steinman MA, Hanlon JT. Managing medications in clinically complex elders: "There's got to be a happy medium." JAMA 2010;304:1592–601.
40. Cooney D, Pascuzzi K. Polypharmacy in the elderly: focus on drug interactions and adherence in hypertension. Clin Geriatr Med 2009;25:221–33.
41. Cramer JA, Roy A, Burrell A, et al. Medication compliance and persistence: terminology and definitions. Value Health 2008;11:44–7.
42. Institute of Medicine (IOM). Initial national priorities for comparative effectiveness research. Washington, DC: The National Academies Press; 2009.
43. Garfinkel D, Mangin D. Feasibility study of a systematic approach for discontinuation of multiple medications in older adults: addressing polypharmacy. Arch Intern Med 2010;170:1648–54.
44. Becker MH, Maiman LA. Sociobehavioral determinants of compliance with health and medical care recommendations. Med Care 1975;13:10–24.

Electronic Prescribing and Other Forms of Technology to Reduce Inappropriate Medication Use and Polypharmacy in Older People: A Review of Current Evidence

Barbara Clyne, BSocSC, MSocSC[a,*],
Marie C. Bradley, PhD, MPharm, MPSI, MPSNI[a,b],
Carmel Hughes, PhD, MRPharmS, MPSNI[b],
Tom Fahey, MSc, MD, DCH, Dobs, MEd Cert, MFPH, FRCGP[a],
Kate L. Lapane, PhD[c]

KEYWORDS

- Polypharmacy • Inappropriate prescribing • Medication use
- Electronic prescribing • Computerized decision support
- Older people

The medication use process includes the following stages: prescribing, dispensing, administering, and monitoring of medications. The prescribing stage is a key target for improving medication-related safety, as prescribing errors are a major source of medication-related problems, such as adverse drug events.[1] Older people are particularly vulnerable to prescribing errors such as inappropriate prescribing, polypharmacy, and adverse drug events.[2] Older people tend to have multiple conditions, with 65% having 2 or more chronic conditions such as diabetes and heart failure,[3] requiring multiple drug treatments. Older people also experience increased sensitivity to medications because of age-related changes in physiology and body composition, which affect pharmacokinetic and pharmacodynamic processes,[4,5] making prescribing

[a] HRB Centre for Primary Care Research, Royal College of Surgeons in Ireland (RCSI), Division of Population Health Science, Beaux Lane House, Lower Mercer Street, Dublin 2, Ireland
[b] School of Pharmacy, Queen's University Belfast, 97 Lisburn Road, Belfast BT9 7BL, UK
[c] Virginia Commonwealth University, Box 98012, 830 East Main Road, Richmond, VA, USA
* Corresponding author.
E-mail address: barbaraclyne@rcsi.ie

Clin Geriatr Med 28 (2012) 301–322
doi:10.1016/j.cger.2012.01.009
0749-0690/12/$ – see front matter © 2012 Elsevier Inc. All rights reserved.

> **Box 1**
> **Key definitions**
>
> **Medication errors:** any preventable event that may cause or lead to inappropriate medication use or patient harm while the medication is in the control of health professional, patient, or consumer.[6]
>
> **Inappropriate Prescribing:** The use of medicines that introduce a greater risk of adverse drug-related events where a safer, as-effective, alternative therapy is available to treat the same condition. It also includes the use of medicines at a higher frequency and for longer than clinically indicated, the use of medicines that have recognized drug-drug interactions, and the underuse of other clinically relevant medications.[2]
>
> **Polypharmacy:** The use of 5 or more medicines.[7]
>
> **Adverse drug events (ADEs):** Any response to a drug that is noxious and unintended.[6]

medications for older people a complex and challenging process. The aim of this review is to provide an overview of the current evidence in relation to the use of technologies to reduce inappropriate medication use in older people, focusing on the prescribing stage (**Box 1**).

BACKGROUND

Inappropriate Prescribing in Older People

Medicines in older people are considered appropriate when they have a clear evidence-based indication, are well tolerated in the majority, and are cost effective. In contrast, medicines that are potentially inappropriate have no clear evidence-based indication, carry a substantially higher risk of adverse side effects, and are not cost effective.[8] Inappropriate prescribing encompasses the use of medicines at a higher frequency and for longer than clinically indicated, the use of medicines that have recognized drug–drug interactions, and the underuse of other clinically relevant medications.[2] Appropriateness in prescribing is generally assessed using either process or outcome measures that are explicit or implicit.[9] Explicit process measures are criterion based and are developed from published reviews, expert opinion, or consensus techniques and usually consist of drugs to be avoided in older people, for example, the Beers criteria[10] and the European Screening Tool of Older Persons' Potentially Inappropriate Prescriptions (STOPP).[11] Implicit approaches are judgment based, compiling patient information and research evidence to assess appropriateness using instruments such as the Medicine Appropriateness Index (MAI).[12] Inappropriate prescribing in older patients is high, with estimates (depending on the criteria used and the cohort under study) ranging from 18% to 48.7% in ambulatory care,[13–15] 25% to 54% in hospitalized patients,[16,17] and 37% to 67% in nursing home residents.[18,19] Inappropriate prescribing in older people can result in increased morbidity, adverse drug events, hospitalizations, and mortality.[9,20,21]

Polypharmacy

Polypharmacy is common in older people. The prevalence of polypharmacy in older people in the United States, defined as the use of 5 or more medicines, was estimated at 7%.[7] Individuals over 65, who account for less than 15% of the US population, consumed 33% of prescription medicines and 40% of over-the-counter medicines.[22] Polypharmacy in older patients has been related to demographic factors, health status, and access to health care,[23] including factors such as white race and education,[24] poorer health, number of health care visits,[25] and multiple providers of health care.[26] Polypharmacy may describe prescribing of many drugs (appropriately) or too many drugs (inappropriately).[27] Despite this, polypharmacy has been associated with negative health outcomes, including adverse drug reactions, poor adherence, inappropriate prescribing, and geriatric syndromes such as urinary incontinence, cognitive impairment, and impaired balance leading to falls.[23] There is a 13% risk of an adverse drug event with the use of 2 medications, but with 5 medications, it increases to 58%[28] and with 7 or more medications, it further increases to 82%.[29]

Health Information Technology and Prescribing in Older People

Many technological applications are currently available in health care, and these can be categorized into 3 broad functional areas: (1) those that enable data storage, management, and retrieval; (2) those that facilitate care from a distance; and (3) those that support clinical decision making.[30] The first 2 categories have more indirect effects on medication use and prescribing and are briefly summarized here. The third category includes the use of electronic prescribing (or e-prescribing) and computerized decision support system (CDSS) technologies and is the main focus of this review.

Data storage, management, and retrieval systems

The use of electronic medical records (EMRs) is core to data storage, management, and retrieval systems. The EMR adoption rate in the United States had increased to 48.3% in ambulatory care by the end of 2009[31] and routine use of EMRs is reported in 7 European countries.[32] EMRs can be used for the digital input, storage, display, retrieval, printing, and sharing of information contained in a patient's health record.[30] A recent study in a hospital setting found EMRs to assist with ascertaining accurate medication history and in reducing medication errors, however, the quality of the data contained in the EMR may be poor.[33] Older people use many health care services and consequently have multiple care providers at the same time. By allowing multiple care providers (usually within an organization) to access a patient's information, EMRs offer the potential to enable providers at the point of care to utilize patient health history to provide better care,[34] and potentially reduce medication errors. However, the capacity to successfully integrate numerous records across health care settings relating to the same older person has not been adequately developed.[35]

Facilitating care from a distance

Telehealth technologies are key applications used in providing care from a distance. Telehealth can be defined as the use of videoconferencing or other telecommunication technologies to enable communication between patients and health care providers separated by geographical distance.[36] It was previously known as telemedicine, and these terms continue to be used interchangeably in the literature.[37] Most European countries report use of telehealth technology; however, this tends to be on a small and experimental level.[32] Telehealth applications are very diverse, ranging from home care for chronic diseases to remote primary care.[37] In particular, these technologies can play a role in the monitoring stage of the medication use process, supporting medication adherence in older people through the use of monitoring and reminders and offering a patient management approach that empowers patients, influences their attitudes and behaviors, and potentially improves their medical conditions.[36,38] It may enhance patient access to health care professionals and is most effective when used to monitor and respond to ongoing patient symptomatology and facilitate information exchange across interdisciplinary teams.

However, the sustainability of telemedicine interventions for the broad spectrum of older patients' issues presents ongoing challenges to telemedicine-delivered care.[39]

Supporting clinical decision making— E-prescribing and CDSS

Electronic prescribing (e-prescribing) is the direct computer-to-computer transmission of prescription information from physician offices to pharmacies. By using a computer or handheld device with e-prescribing software, prescribers access patient prescription benefit information and patient medication history and electronically direct prescriptions to a patient's pharmacy of choice.[40] By the end of 2010, about 34% of office-based practices in the United States were using some variant of this technology.[41] In the United States, federal initiatives have stimulated increases in e-prescribing.[42] In the United States, a key feature of e-prescribing is the bidirectional flow of information from physician office to pharmacy and back. The technology provides physicians with a system to track patient refill histories, streamline the administration of patient records, check for drug conflicts, and facilitate better communication between pharmacies and physician offices.[43] E-prescribing is expected to assist in both increasing efficiency and reducing medication errors.[44–46]

Adoption in Europe has been slower, however, with a full e-prescribing process used routinely in just 4 countries, namely, Denmark, Estonia, Iceland, and Sweden.[32] It should be remembered that the obstacles to the successful implementation of e-prescribing software in physician office practices are non-trivial and real and include the financial costs and opportunity costs (personnel and time) of implementation, lack of standardized software, and lack of systematic evidence of effectiveness.[47] Despite the challenges, e-prescribing will take on a greater role in patient management in general.[42] Although time-in-motion studies point to increased time to actually write e-prescriptions,[48] recent studies show that physicians and staff identify efficiencies gained by minimizing calls from pharmacy relating to prescription choices not being on formulary, reduced time spent on prior authorizations, reduced time spent processing refills, and overall better workflow because of decreased time spent performing refill requests.[49,50]

Medication errors may be reduced by the use of CDSS in e-prescribing systems.[51] CDSSs are information systems designed to improve clinical decision making. Characteristics of individual patients are matched to a computerized knowledge base, and software algorithms generate patient-specific recommendations that can be delivered to the clinician through the EMR, by pager, or through printouts placed in a patient's paper chart.[52] E-prescribing systems can also integrate/interface with EMRs or be an element of a broader computerized provider/physician order entry (CPOE) system.[30] CPOE systems are computer applications that allow direct, electronic entry of orders for medications, laboratory, radiology, referral, and procedures.[53] The use of e-prescribing within, or in conjunction with, these systems provides the ability to check automatically for dose errors and drug–drug/drug–disease interactions as well as provide warnings and information to enable the prescriber to make changes at the time of prescribing[54]; it has shown the potential for changing professional practice, particularly with regard to drug ordering.[52,55–58] E-prescribing has shown promise in tackling many of the problems associated with the use of medications in older people.[5] However, much of the literature in the area has focused on general populations or in just 1 setting (eg, in-patient care), and there has been less focus on the effectiveness of these technologies in older people. We undertook a comprehensive literature search as described in **Box 2** to identify studies pertaining to the use of the technologies described above, specifically in older people.

Box 2
Search strategy

PubMed, EMBASE, and the Cochrane Database of Systematic Reviews databases were searched to identify articles on e-prescribing and other technology to improve inappropriate medication use and polypharmacy using a combination of the following MeSH terms and key words: inappropriate prescribing; polypharmacy; drug therapy; electronic prescribing; medication errors; decision support systems, clinical; medical order entry systems; alerts; health informatics; aged; elderly; intervention studies; Controlled Clinical Trials as Topic.

Articles in English that measured changes in inappropriate prescribing and/or polypharmacy in older people (aged 65 years of age and older) using e-prescribing or other technology were included. Articles were excluded where it was clear from title/abstract review that they did not relate to older people, changes in inappropriate prescribing, and/or polypharmacy or e-prescribing or other technology. Articles were not excluded on the basis of methodology (eg, not a randomized, controlled trial). Articles were categorized into ambulatory care, hospital/in-patient care, and long-term care and categorized according to a generally accepted hierarchy of evidence, with experimental studies at the highest level of evidence. Outcomes were assessed in terms of process (medication-related) measures and patient outcomes, such as morbidity.

OVERVIEW OF CURRENT EVIDENCE FOR E-PRESCRIBING AND OTHER FORMS OF TECHNOLOGY TO REDUCE INAPPROPRIATE MEDICATION USE AND POLYPHARMACY IN OLDER PEOPLE
Ambulatory Care

E-prescribing and CDSS style interventions have the potential to improve outcomes in ambulatory care.[59,60] From our literature search we identified 6 studies conducted in ambulatory care that examined the use of e-prescribing and CDSS to reduce polypharmacy and inappropriate prescribing in older people. A summary of the studies can be seen in **Table 1**.

A cluster randomized, controlled trial (RCT) assessed a CDSS intervention that involved providing access to a complete drug profile (of all current and past prescriptions) through a dedicated computer link between the electronic patient chart and a drug-insurance program.[61] When a prescribing problem was identified by the CDSS software, the physician received an alert that identified the nature of the problem, possible consequences, and alternative therapy. The study found that the intervention reduced prescriptions for new inappropriate drugs in the intervention group, but had no significant impact on the discontinuation of pre-existing inappropriate prescriptions. The effectiveness of the intervention may have been influenced by unforeseen factors, including an increase in co-payments for prescription drugs during the study period and frequent hardware/software failure during early stages of the trial.

Delivering prescribing alerts at the pharmacy level was found to be effective in another RCT.[62] The pharmacist was notified via a medication alert generated from the pharmacy information management system when patients in the intervention group received a new inappropriate prescription. Prescription labels failed to print until the pharmacist had intervened. Alternative therapy options were discussed with the prescriber via telephone. The primary outcome in this study was the number of inappropriate medications dispensed. This was estimated at 1.8% for the intervention group compared with 2.2% in the usual care group. The authors highlight the modest difference in numbers of dispensing between groups as evidence of the challenging nature of modifying prescriber behavior, even in the context of an intervention that has widespread institutional and prescriber support.

Table 1
Characteristics of studies in ambulatory care

Reference (Country)	Study Design (N)	Intervention(s)	Outcomes
Tamblyn, et al,[61] 2003 (Canada)	Cluster RCT (12,560)	Computerized age-specific pop-up alerts (≥66 years of age) for 159 prescribing problems inc. Drug-disease interactions, drug-drug interactions, drug-age interactions and drug duplication. Alert identifies nature of the problem, possible consequences and alternative therapy	**P:** Number of new PIP per 1000 visits was significantly lower (18%) in the CDS group than in the control group (RR, 0.82; 95% CI, 0.69–0.98), but differences between the groups in the rate of discontinuation of PIP were significant only for therapeutic duplication by the study physician and another physician (RR, 1.66; 95% CI, 0.99–2.79) and drug interactions caused by prescriptions written by the study physician (RR, 2.15; 95% CI, 0.98–4.70).
Raebel et al,[62] 2007 (US)	RCT (59,680)	Age-specific alerts for pharmacists when a patient age 65 and older was newly prescribed 1 of 11 potentially inappropriate medications. Pharmacist contacts prescriber, suggesting alternative	**P:** 1.8% intervention group patients were newly dispensed prescriptions for targeted medications versus 2.2% in usual care group patients (P = .002). Significant decrease in dispensing of amitriptyline and diazepam.
Weber et al,[63] 2007 (US)	RCT (620)	Pharmacist reviewed patient charts, message was sent to prescriber via EMR alerting them that the patient was at risk for falls and made patient recommendations re: specific medications or dosing	**P:** The intervention did not reduce the total number of medications. There was a significant negative relationship between the intervention and the total number of medications started during the intervention period (P<.01) and the total number of psychoactive medications (P<.05). **PT:** The impact on falls was mixed; with intervention group 0.38 times as likely to have had 1 or more fall-related diagnosis (P<.01) over study period.
Smith et al,[64] 2006 (US)	Interrupted time series (450,000)	Computerized drug-specific alerts with suggested alternative medication for certain long-acting benzodiazepines and TCAs	**P:** Reduction in nonpreferred drugs of 5.1 prescriptions per 10,000, P = .004, a 22% relative decrease from before alert implementation.

Simon et al,[65] 2006 (US)	Interrupted time series (239 physicians, 50,924 patients)	Follow-up study in which computerized age-specific alerts (≥65 years of age) replaced drug-specific alerts, occurring at the time of prescribing for targeted potentially inappropriate medication (eg, TCAs, long-acting benzodiazepines) with suggested alternative medication and academic detailing	**P:** Age-specific alerts resulted in a continuation of the effects of the drug-specific alerts without measurable additional effect ($P = .75$ for level change), but the age-specific alerts led to fewer false-positive alerts for clinicians. Group academic detailing did not enhance the effect of the alerts.
Monane,[66] 1998 (US)	Cohort study (23,269)	Online computerized drug utilization review database alerts pharmacists to inappropriate drug use, pharmacist contacts prescriber to discuss principles of geriatric pharmacology and alternatives	**P:** A total of 24,266 recommendations were made. Rate of change to a more appropriate therapeutic agent was 24% but ranged from 40% for long half-life benzodiazepines to 2% to 7% for drugs that theoretically were contraindicated by patients' self-reported history.

Abbreviations: P, process (medication-related outcomes); PIP, potentially inappropriate prescribing; PT, patient-related outcomes.

An EMR-based intervention to reduce overall medication use, psychoactive medication use, and the occurrence of falls failed to yield positive results.[63] A standardized medication review was conducted by a pharmacist, and a message was sent to the prescriber via the EMR, alerting them that the patient was at risk of falls and making recommendations with regard to specific medications or dosing. The intervention did not reduce the total number of medications, but there was a significant negative relationship between the intervention and the total number of medications started during the intervention period and the total number of psychoactive medications. Despite this, the findings were limited by the small sample size.

A study by Smith and coworkers[64] integrated drug-specific alerts into an existing CPOE system, alerting clinicians to preferred alternative medications when they ordered certain long-acting benzodiazepines and tertiary amine tricyclic antidepressants (TCAs). A 22% relative decrease in the use of non-preferred medications after the intervention implementation, when compared with the month before alert implementation, was reported. A follow-up interrupted time series study in the same population found no additional significant effects after changing the drug-specific alerts to age-specific alerts (≥65 years of age). However, there was a decrease in the number of false-positive alerts (ie, alerts received when prescribing a medication that was not contraindicated for their age for those aged <65).[65] These 2 studies may have limited generalizability, as they were conducted in a Health Maintenance Organization with several years' experience in the use of CPOE and CDSS; therefore, participants may have been more receptive to these alerts than clinicians elsewhere.

A computerized drug utilization review was found to improve prescribing in a study by Monane and colleagues[66] As part of the intervention, pharmacists were instructed how to use the drug utilization review program. When a potentially inappropriate medication was ordered, the computer sent a message to the pharmacist who subsequently called the physician to discuss the medication and possible therapeutic alternatives. The study findings showed improved prescribing patterns, with a 24% rate of change to a more appropriate therapeutic agent. The reasons physicians gave for not changing included not seeing the intervention as applicable to the patient, disagreeing with intervention, or seeing the intervention as inconvenient for the patient and patient preference. The authors noted that this study may have underestimated the extent of the problem and overestimated the potential benefit of the intervention, as it was based on mail-service prescriptions and did not include retail pharmacies.

Hospital/In-Patient Care

E-prescribing and CPOE systems can have a positive impact on care in the hospital setting.[67] We identified 4 studies in our literature search that looked at the use of e-prescribing and CDSS to reduce polypharmacy and inappropriate prescribing in older people in a hospital setting. A summary of the studies can be seen in **Table 2**.

Terrell and colleagues[68] integrated CDSS into the existing CPOE system in an emergency department. Alerts appeared when the physician tried to order one of the targeted medications and offered alternatives. There was a significant decrease in the proportion of all prescribed medications that were inappropriate from 5.4% to 3.4% postintervention. However, the study targeted a small sample of academic physicians and residents; thus, findings may not be generalizable to other providers or health care settings.

Peterson and coworkers[69] aimed to improve psychotropic drug selection among hospitalized older people by integrating CDSS into the existing CPOE system in the form of geriatric specific default dosages for targeted medications and suggested

Table 2
Characteristics of studies in hospital care

Reference	Study Design (N)	Intervention(s)	Outcomes
Terrell et al,[68] 2009 (US)	RCT (63)	Age-specific alerts occurring at the time of prescribing in ED for 1 of 9 potentially inappropriate medications with recommended alternatives	**P:** Intervention physicians prescribed 1 or more inappropriate medications during 2.6% of ED visits by seniors, compared with 3.9% of visits managed by control physicians ($P = .02$; OR $= 0.55$; 95% CI, 0.34–0.89). The proportion of all prescribed medications that were inappropriate significantly decreased from 5.4% to 3.4%.
Peterson et al,[69] 2005 (US)	Interrupted time series (3718)	Age-specific dosing suggestions and alternatives when physician ordered 1 of 12 psychotropic medications known to be poorly tolerated/higher risk in older people	**P:** The intervention increased the prescription of the recommended daily dose (29% vs 19%; $P<.001$), reduced the incidence of 10-fold dosing (2.8% vs 5.0%; $P<.001$), and reduced the prescription of nonrecommended drugs (10.8% vs 7.6% of total orders; $P<.001$). **PT:** Patients in the intervention cohort had a lower in-hospital fall rate (0.28 vs 0.64 falls per 100 patient-days; $P = .001$). No effect on hospital length of stay or days of altered mental status was found.
Agostini et al,[70] 2007 (US)	Before/after (24,509)	Computer-based reminder directing clinicians to prescribe a nonpharmacologic sleep protocol, to minimize the potential for harm with diphenhydramine and diazepam use by choosing an alternative medication (trazodone or lorazepam), or both	**P:** Prescribing of sedative-hypnotics decreased from 18% in patients preintervention to 15% postintervention (OR, 0.82; 95% CI, 0.76–0.87), an 18% risk reduction. Ninety-five percent of patients were successfully directed to a safer sedative-hypnotic drug or a nonpharmacologic sleep protocol.
Mattison et al,[71] 2010 (US)	Before/after	Drug-specific warning system within CPOE system that alerted ordering prescriber when ordering one of the targeted medicines and advised alternative medication or dose reduction.	**P:** The mean rate of ordering medications that were not recommended decreased from 11.56 (SE $= 0.36$) to 9.94 (SE $= 0.12$) orders per day after the implementation of a CPOE warning system (difference, 1.62 [0.33]; P-value $.001$), with no evidence that the effect waned over time.

Abbreviations: ED, emergency department; P, Process (medication-related outcomes); PT, patient-related outcomes.

alternatives. The study findings showed that the intervention increased the prescription of recommended doses (29% vs 19%), reduced the prescription of nonrecommended drugs (10.8% vs 7.6% of total orders), and was associated with fewer inpatient falls (0.28 vs 0.64 falls per 100 patient-days). No effect on hospital length of stay or days of altered mental status was found. The lack of randomization in this study was a limitation.

Agostini and colleagues[70] aimed to improve the prescribing of 4 sedative-hypnotic medications via integrating CDSS into an existing CPOE system. When a physician ordered any of the targeted medications, reminder screens appeared on the computer system to check the indication and offer educational reminders about the potential adverse effects, recommendations for appropriate nonpharmacologic and sedative-hypnotic medication, and dosing advice. The study findings were positive, with an 18% risk reduction for prescribing of sedative-hypnotics postintervention. The study hospital had a restricted formulary including only 4 sedative-hypnotic medications; therefore, the findings of this study may not be directly applicable to hospitals with different formularies.

Drug-specific alerts with alternative medications or dose reductions were implemented into an existing CPOE system.[71] The alert was activated when one of the targeted medications was ordered by the physician and alternatives were offered. The study findings showed that CPOE with CDSS did reduce orders for nonrecommended medications from a mean (standard error, SE) of 11.56 (0.36) to 9.94 (0.12) orders per day after the implementation of a CPOE warning system (difference, 1.62 [0.33]; $P = .001$), with no evidence that the effect waned over time. The study could not determine whether ADEs were prevented by the use of the CDSS.

Nursing Home Care

Nursing homes have been slow to integrate CDSS and CPOE systems into their normal work flow[72] even though some studies have found them to be acceptable and feasible.[73–76] Four studies related to the use of CDSS and CPOE in the nursing home setting were identified, and a summary of these is presented in **Table 3**.

A study by Gurwitz and coworkers[77] assessed the effect of CPOE with CDSS on adverse drug events in 2 large long-term care facilities. The CDSS was implemented into the existing CPOE system in the facilities. Possible drug-related incidents were presented to 2 physicians who determined if an ADE was present, the severity of the event, and if the event was preventable. The study findings showed that CPOE with CDSS did not reduce the adverse drug event rate or preventable adverse drug event rate in the long-term care setting. The adjusted odds ratio for all adverse drug events in intervention units versus control units was 1.06 (95% confidence interval [CI], 0.92–1.23). The authors identified various limiting factors that may have contributed to the null results such as alert burden (>50% of the alerts were deemed unnecessary, and this may have been related to the fact that the CPOE system was unable to calculate total daily dose), limited scope of the alerts (41 alerts, which targeted a minority of ADEs identified in the study), and the need to more fully integrate clinical and laboratory information.

A similar RCT investigated the use of CPOE with CDSS and its effect on the appropriateness of prescribing for residents with renal insufficiency in a single long-term care facility. CDSS alerts for adjusting the dose and frequency of medication orders for residents were displayed to prescribers in the intervention units and hidden but tracked in control units. The proportion of appropriate final drug orders was significantly higher in the intervention units compared with control units. This study was limited by the possibility of contamination, as the physicians operating in

Table 3
Characteristics of studies in nursing home care

Reference	Study Design (N)	Intervention(s)	Outcomes
Gurwitz et al,[77] 2008 (US)	Cluster RCT (1,118)	Thirty-nine clinical decision support criteria and 41 corresponding alerts were developed based on adverse drug events identified from previous research and a standard pharmaceutical drug interaction database and integrated into the existing CPOE system in 2 long-term care settings. The CDSS appeared in the form of a pop-up box in real time when the drug order was entered by physician.	P: Adverse drug events that may have resulted from medication errors (eg, errors in ordering, dispensing, administration and monitoring) or from adverse drug reactions in which there was no error. CPOE with CDSS did not reduce the adverse drug event rate or preventable adverse drug event rate in the long-term care setting. Comparing intervention and control units, the adjusted rate ratios were 1.06 (95% CI, 0.92–1.23) for all adverse drug events and 1.02 (95% CI, 0.81–1.30) for preventable adverse drug events.
Field et al,[78] 2009 (Canada)	Cluster RCT (833)	Conducted in a single long-term care facility among 833 residents over 12 months. A list of 62 drugs that may have needed dose or frequency adjustments was compiled and alerts related to the prescribing of these agents for residents with renal insufficiency were displayed to prescribers in the intervention units and hidden but tracked in control units. Four types of alerts were developed.	P: The proportion of final drug orders that were appropriate was significantly higher in the intervention units (RR, 1.2; 95% CI, 1.0–1.4). The proportions of dose alerts for which the final drug orders were appropriate were similar between the intervention and control units (RR, 0.95; 95% CI, 0.83, 1.1).

(continued on next page)

Table 3
(continued)

Reference	Study Design (N)	Intervention(s)	Outcomes
Colon-Emeric et al,[72] 2009 (US)	Before/after (265)	Development and pilot testing (to examine feasibility and acceptance) of computerized order entry algorithms for geriatric problems in nursing homes among 42 Veteran's Affairs nursing home providers. Computerized order entry algorithms based on clinical practice guidelines were developed. These were presented to physicians at the time of prescribing on a single screen and provided an array of diagnostic and treatment options and means to communicate with the interdisciplinary team.	P: Use was infrequent and varied according to condition: falls (73.0%), fever (9.0%), pneumonia (8.0%), urinary tract infection (7.0%), and osteoporosis (3.0%). PT: In subjects with falls, trends for improvements in quality measures were observed for 6 of the 9 measures. Little improvement was observed in the other conditions There was no change in resource utilization.
Judge et al,[79] 2006 (US)	Study within a cluster RCT (445)	Thirty-nine clinical decision support criteria and 41 corresponding alerts were developed and integrated into the existing CPOE system in 2 long-term care settings. This study assessed prescribers' responses to alerts generated by a CDSS system.	P: A total of 47,997 medication orders were entered through the CPOE system and 9,414 alerts were triggered. Prescribers who received alerts were only slightly more likely to take an appropriate action (RR, 1.11; 95% CI, 1.00, 1.22).

Abbreviations: P, process (medication-related outcomes); PT, patient-related outcomes.

intervention units also worked in control units, and their prescribing practices in the intervention groups may have influenced the care given in the control units. This study found that clinical decision support provided for physicians prescribing medications for long-term care residents (with renal insufficiency) can improve care and that CDSS implemented within a commercial CPOE system was successful and had capacity for further linkage.[78]

A study by Judge et al,[79] set within the RCT described above,[77] assessed prescribers' responses to alerts generated by a CDSS system. The frequency of drug orders, associated with various alerts, was assessed. Overall prescribers who received the alerts were only slightly more likely to pursue an appropriate action. Alerts related to prescriptions for warfarin or central nervous system side effects were more likely to lead to an appropriate action. The authors concluded that the low rate of response to the alerts triggered by the CDSS suggested that further adjustments to the system were necessary.

A study investigating the development and pilot testing of computerized order entry algorithms for geriatric problems in Veterans' Affairs (VA) nursing homes found infrequent and varied use of computerized order entry algorithm. However, CPOE was used in 73% of falls cases, and some improvements were noted in quality measures related to these incidents. This study was limited by the fact that it was carried out at VA nursing homes; therefore, the findings may not be generalizable to community nursing homes. VA nursing homes have more on-site providers and an electronic order medical record system, which may not be available in community nursing homes. The authors concluded that this technology exhibited potential promise for improving clinical practice guideline use in nursing homes, but further modifications to adapt to the community nursing home system and to prompt use for chronic conditions was needed.[72]

Other studies in the nursing home sector that did not specifically focus on the prescribing stage of medication use, are complimentary to this discussion—The Geriatric Risk Assessment MedGuide (GRAM) study and the Fleetwood study are 2 such studies. GRAM[80] was an RCT that examined the extent to which the use of a clinical informatics tool that implemented prospective monitoring plans reduced the incidence of potential delirium, falls, hospitalizations caused by adverse drug events, and mortality among 25 nursing homes. The intervention involved the pharmacies generating GRAM reports to identify medications that may cause, aggravate, or contribute to common or serious geriatric problems and automated monitoring plans to prospectively detect serious geriatric problems that may have been caused by medications. Overall, this study found that newly admitted residents in intervention homes experienced a significantly lower rate of potential delirium onset than those in usual care homes. Lower rates of overall hospitalization and mortality were reported, but these findings did not reach statistical significance. The intervention had no effect on falls. The positive effects of the intervention were not seen in longer stay residents, although it had been hypothesized that because of the nature of the intervention, the effect would be stronger in new admissions.

The Fleetwood study used a before-and-after design with a non-randomized comparison group and utilized health information technology to improve communication and implement the Fleetwood Model of pharmaceutical care. This was performed by dispensing and consultant pharmacists and incorporated prospective reviews, direct communication with the prescribers, and formalized pharmaceutical care planning in patients at highest risk for medication-related problems. It was conducted in 25 nursing homes in North Carolina. Residents in the intervention had similar hospitalization rates, hospitalizations owing to potential adverse drug events, and mortality rates as residents in the usual care homes. With respect to the use of potentially inappropriate medications, the decline of use of these medications appeared earlier in the intervention homes relative to the usual care homes, but differences did not reach statistical significance (adjusted Hazard Rate=0.86; 95% CI: 0.65–1.12).[81]

DISCUSSION
Summary of Main Findings—Process Measures

This review has provided an overview of the current evidence in relation to the use of e-prescribing and CDSS technology to reduce inappropriate prescribing and polypharmacy in older people. Eleven of the 14 studies identified reported positive outcomes for the use of e-prescribing and CDSS in lowering rates of inappropriate prescribing and polypharmacy. However, the magnitude of effect sizes reported for interventions varied according to study design and setting, and some studies focused on different drug classes.

In ambulatory care, 4 studies reported positive outcomes. Both RCT designs described favorable outcomes. Tamblyn and colleagues[61] reduced the inappropriate prescription rate by 18%, whereas Raebel and coworkers[62] reported that just 1.8% of intervention group patients received a newly dispensed inappropriate prescription compared with 2.2% in usual care, a smaller magnitude of effect but relevant nonetheless. One study using an interrupted time series design found a 22% relative decrease in the exposure of older people to certain benzodiazepines and TCAs when drug-specific alerts were implemented.[64] In a follow-up to this study, Simon et al[65] found that changing drug-specific alerts to age-specific alerts produced no additional effect on the rates of inappropriate prescribing. The only cohort study (which is low on the hierarchy of research design) included in this review also showed positive outcomes, reporting a rate of change to a more appropriate therapeutic agent of 24%. An RCT by Weber and coworkers[63] was the only study conducted in the ambulatory care setting to report a negative finding. In that study, the introduction of pharmacist-initiated EMR alerts did not reduce the overall number of medications; however, this was possibly related to the small sample size.

All studies conducted in hospital or in-patient settings showed positive outcomes. However, the magnitude of the findings again varied by study design and intervention type. The only RCT[68] included found that the proportion of inappropriate prescriptions reduced from 5.4% to 3.4% overall, whereas an interrupted time series study found a reduction in the prescription of inappropriate prescriptions from 10.8% to 7.6%.[69] For sedative-hypnotic prescribing, one study reported an 18% risk reduction after intervention,[70] whereas a similar study found the mean rate of ordering of nonrecommended medications decreased from 11.56 to 9.94 orders per day after intervention.[71]

In the nursing home sector, 3 studies reported positive outcomes. Judge and colleagues[79] reported a small positive effect in 1 RCT with prescribers in the intervention group only slightly more likely to pursue an appropriate action. Similarly, a cluster RCT found appropriate drug orders were higher in intervention units than control.[78] The study by Gurwitz and colleagues[77] did not show favorable benefits of CPOE with CDSS on adverse drug events in the long-term care setting; however, it is important to recognize that adverse drug events are less common than inappropriate drug orders, so differences may be more difficult to detect. The need to increase the use of CPOE with CDSS to a broader range of drug safety issues is, therefore, apparent.

In all but one study across all 3 settings, alternative agents were offered to the prescriber to accept, whether at the point of prescribing directly or more indirectly via pharmacist review. One of the studies with negative findings, Gurwitz and coworkers[77] did not offer alternative agents for prescribers to accept, indicating that drug-specific alerts with alternative therapy advice may be important elements of successful interventions to improve inappropriate prescribing.

Summary of Main Findings—Patient Outcomes

Although some promising results were reported in this review, which suggested that e-prescribing and CDSS style interventions may be successful in improving appropriate prescribing and polypharmacy, the clinical impact of this is not known. Few studies in this review examined the effect of the interventions on patient outcomes such as hospitalizations, morbidity, and mortality, which limited the interpretation of such interventions. In a study in which a pharmacist inserted alerts into EMRs in ambulatory care, a mixed effect on the incidence of falls was reported, with the intervention group 0.38 times as likely to have had 1 or more fall-related diagnosis.[63] Peterson and coworkers[69] reported a lower in-hospital fall rate for those in the CDSS intervention group but noted no effect on hospital length of stay or days of altered mental status. Health information technology in nursing home settings has the potential to be successful if specific recommendations for ordering[78] or monitoring[80] are provided; however, to date, the impact on patient outcomes appears minimal.[81]

Challenges to Adoption of E-Prescribing and Other Technologies

Despite the vast heterogeneity in the included studies in terms of intervention types, health care settings, and study designs, the use of health information technology, including e-prescribing with CPOE and CDSS, has demonstrated some potential in improving appropriate, safe, and effective prescribing in all the care settings described. However, widespread diffusion of these interventions has not occurred, and it would appear that there are various obstacles that need to be surmounted before significant effects can be seen.

The attitudes of health care professionals can be a significant factor in the acceptance and efficiency of use of health information technology in practice[82] and, as Raebel and colleagues[62] note, changing prescriber behavior can be very difficult. While physicians and pharmacists generally report being satisfied with e-prescribing systems and see the systems as having a positive impact on the safety of their prescribing practices,[83–86] a number of obstacles to the successful implementation of such systems have been reported. These include a lack of trust in technology, the associated costs of implementation, a lack of integration of systems and standards, lack of systematic evidence of effectiveness, and the potential for new patient safety issues to arise, such as "juxtaposition error," when an item near the one actually desired is clicked by mistake.[47,87–90]

Costs are a particularly salient concern in the nursing home setting. Although studies have found feasible and effective approaches to reducing harm owing to medication use among nursing home residents, how to stimulate adoption and who would pay for this in the US context has yet to be determined. In the years since the Institute of Medicine report calling for nursing homes to implement and use clinical information systems to support clinical practice,[91] adoption of health information technology in nursing homes has been slow.[92] Indeed, 1% or less of skilled nursing facilities have electronic health records used for clinical processes.[93] Recent research suggests that nursing homes are using technology for improving care processes[94] and indeed some tools are being designed specifically for this purpose.[95] One such nursing home chain, HCR Manor Care, has increased its use of health information technology by investing in more than 10,000 personal computers as well as expansion of facilities.[96]

Another significant barrier to the adoption and use of e-prescribing and CDSS systems centers on electronic alerts. Health care professionals recognize the positive impact that alerts can have on patient safety[43,97]; however, there is a problematic lack of acceptance of alerts in clinical systems.[98] It has been estimated that anywhere between 49% and 96% of alerts are overridden or ignored.[99] Alerts are overridden because of a range of factors, including unsuitable content of alerts, excessive frequency of alerts, and alerts causing unwarranted disruption to the prescriber's workflow, as was noted in the study by Gurwitz and colleagues.[77,100] Alerts are more likely to be well received if they are focused on highly critical information, can be trusted to provide high accuracy, and are designed to promote efficient information retrieval.[101] Other strategies recommended by physicians for the improvement of e-prescribing include the simplification of drug choice and cancellation of e-prescriptions.[86]

Patients themselves tend to be largely absent from discussions on the use of technology in prescribing, and less research has been conducted in this area. A recent study in Sweden found patients generally report a positive attitude toward e-prescriptions and electronic storing of prescriptions. A majority affirmed that such systems were safe, created benefits, and promoted faster dispensing. However, attitudes differ according to age, with younger age groups having the most positive attitudes and the older age groups having the least positive attitudes.[102] A survey of older patients in the United States found that e-prescribing technology solutions may provide opportunities for earlier and enhanced communication between geriatric patients and their clinicians about their medications, but generally, older patients may require more education to appreciate the value of e-prescribing.[103]

Comparison with Existing Literature

Previous reviews on improving prescribing in older populations have suggested (in line with our findings) that computerized decision support interventions may be effective in improving prescribing practices.[9,104–106]

Limitations

This review has a number of shortcomings. First, this review was not conducted systematically. It was a narrative review, and a meta-analysis was not conducted because of the level of heterogeneity among the studies. The studies included differed in terms of study design, the interventions delivered, the intensity and duration of interventions, and the outcomes measured, and it was difficult to tease out the exact components of the interventions that were most successful.

Future Research

Future research should continue to focus on evaluating the use of e-prescribing and other technologies to reduce inappropriate prescribing and polypharmacy in older people. It would appear that more formal rigorous investigations into these systems are required to enhance patient safety in all settings. More emphasis on the effect of interventions on patient-centered outcomes such as morbidity, mortality, and hospitalizations is needed. The barriers and obstacles to successful implementation of CDSS- and CPOE-type interventions, such as alert fatigue, need to be more fully investigated and workable solutions developed. Increasing the success of these interventions requires focused strategies to overcome the barriers to implementation.

SUMMARY

This review provided an overview of the current evidence in relation to the use of e-prescribing and other forms of technology, such as CDSS, to reduce inappropriate prescribing in older people. The evidence indicates that various types of e-prescribing and CDSS interventions have the potential to reduce inappropriate prescribing and polypharmacy in older people, but the magnitude of their effect varies according to study design and setting. There was significant heterogeneity in the studies reported in terms of study designs, intervention design, patient settings, and outcome measures with patient outcomes seldom reported. Widespread diffusion of these interventions has not occurred in any of the health care settings examined. Overall, health care providers report being satisfied with e-prescribing systems and see the systems as having a positive impact on the safety of their prescribing practices, yet the problem of overriding or ignoring alerts persists. The problem of large numbers of inaccurate and insignificant alerts and this issue, along with the other barriers that have been identified, warrant further investigation.

REFERENCES

1. Barber N, Rawlins M, Dean Franklin B. Reducing prescribing error: competence, control, and culture. Qual Saf Health Care 2003;12(Suppl 1):i29–i32.
2. Gallagher P, Barry P, O'Mahony D. Inappropriate prescribing in the elderly. J Clin Pharm Ther 2007;32(2):113–21.
3. Wolff JL, Starfield B, Anderson G. Prevalence, expenditures, and complications of multiple chronic conditions in the elderly. Arch Intern Med 2002;162(20):2269–76.
4. Mangoni A, Jackson S. Age-related changes in pharmacokinetics and pharmaco-dynamics: basic principles and practical applications. Br J Clin Pharmacol 2003;57: 6–14.
5. Milton JC, Hill-Smith I, Jackson SH. Prescribing for older people. BMJ 2008; 336(7644):606–9.
6. Smith J. Building a safer national health system for patients: improving medication safety. London Department of Health, 2004.
7. Kaufman DW, Kelly JP, Rosenberg L, et al. Recent patterns of medication use in the ambulatory adult population of the United States. JAMA 2002;287(3):337–44.
8. O' Mahony D, Gallagher PF. Inappropriate prescribing in the older population: need for new criteria. Age Ageing 2008;37(2):138–41.
9. Spinewine A, Schmader K, Barber N, et al. Appropriate prescribing in elderly people: how well can it be measured and optimised? Lancet 2007;370:173–84.
10. Fick DM, Cooper JW, Wade WE, et al. Updating the Beers criteria for potentially inappropriate medication use in older adults: results of a US consensus panel of experts. Arch Intern Med 2003;163(22):2716–24.
11. Gallagher P, Ryan C, Byrne S, et al. STOPP (Screening Tool of Older Person's Prescriptions) and START (Screening Tool to Alert doctors to Right Treatment). Consensus validation. Int J Clin Pharmacol Ther 2008;46(2):72–83.
12. Hanlon JT, Schmader KE, Samsa GP, et al. A method for assessing drug therapy appropriateness. J Clin Epidemiol 1992;45(10):1045–51.
13. Brekke M, Rognstad S, Straand J, et al. Pharmacologically inappropriate prescriptions for elderly patients in general practice: How common? Scand J Prim Health Care 2008;26(2):80–5.
14. Roughead EE, Anderson B, Gilbert AL. Potentially inappropriate prescribing among Australian veterans and war widows/widowers. Intern Med J 2007;37(6):402–5.

15. Buck MD, Atreja A, Brunker CP, J et al. Potentially inappropriate medication prescribing in outpatient practices: prevalence and patient characteristics based on electronic health records. Am J Geriatr Pharmacother 2009;7(2):84–92.

16. Radoscaronevi N, Gantumur M, Vlahović-Palcevski V, et al. Potentially inappropriate prescribing to hospitalised patients. Pharmacoepidemiol Drug Saf 2008;17(7): 733–7.

17. Conejos Miquel MD, Sánchez Cuervo M, Delgado Silveira E, et al. Potentially inappropriate drug prescription in older subjects across health care settings. Eur Geriatric Med 2010;1(1):9.

18. Barnett K, McCowan C, Evans JMM, et al. Prevalence and outcomes of potentially inappropriate medicines use in the elderly: cohort study stratified by residence in nursing home or in the community. BMJ Qual Saf 2011;20:275–81.

19. Byrne S, O Mahony D, Hughes CM, et al. An evaluation of the inappropriate prescribing in older residents in long term care in the greater Cork and Northern Ireland regions using the STOPP and Beers criteria. Dublin: Centre for ageing research and development in Ireland (CARDI); 2011.

20. Lau DT, Kasper JD, Potter DE, et al. Hospitalization and death associated with potentially inappropriate medication prescriptions among elderly nursing home residents. Arch Intern Med 2005;165(1):68–74.

21. Lin HY, Liao CC, Cheng SH, et al. Association of potentially inappropriate medication use with adverse outcomes in ambulatory elderly patients with chronic diseases: experience in a Taiwanese medical setting. Drugs Aging 2008;25(1):49–59.

22. Werder SF, SH P. Managing polypharmacy. Walking the fine line between help and harm. Curr Psychiatry 2003;2(2):24–36.

23. Hajjar ER, Cafiero AC, Hanlon JT. Polypharmacy in elderly patients. Am J Geriatr Pharmacother 2007;5(4):345–51.

24. Fillenbaum GG, Horner RD, Hanlon JT, et al. Factors predicting change in prescription and nonprescription drug use in a community-residing black and white elderly population. J Clin Epidemiol 1996;49(5):587–93.

25. Jorgensen T, Johansson S, Kennerfalk A, et al. Prescription drug use, diagnoses, and healthcare utilization among the elderly. Ann Pharmacother 2001;35(9):1004–9.

26. Espino DV, Lichtenstein MJ, Hazuda HP, et al. Correlates of prescription and over-the-counter medication usage among older Mexican Americans: the Hispanic EPESE study. Established Population for the epidemiologic study of the elderly. J Am Geriatr Soc 1998;46(10):1228–34.

27. Aronson JK. In defence of polypharmacy. Br J Clin Pharmacol 2004;57(2):119–20.

28. Fulton MM, Riley Allen E. Polypharmacy in the elderly: a literature review. J Am Acad Nurse Practit 2005;17(4):123–32.

29. Prybys KM. Polypharmacy in the elderly: clinical challenges in emergency Practice. Part 1: Overview, etiology and drug interactions. Emerg Med Reports 2002;23(11): 145–53.

30. Black AD, Car J, Pagliari C, et al. The impact of eHealth on the quality and safety of health care: a systematic overview. PLoS Med 2011;8(1):e1000387.

31. CDC. Electronic Medical Record/Electronic Health Record Systems of Office-based Physicians: United States, 2009 and Preliminary 2010 State Estimates. Available at: http://wwwcdcgov/nchs/data/hestat/emr_ehr_09/emr_ehr_09htm. Accessed August 31, 2011.

32. Stroetmann KA, Artmann J, Stroetmann VN, et al. European countries on their journey towards national eHealth infrastructures: European Commision Information Society, 2011.

33. Moore P, Armitage G, Wright J, et al. Medicines reconciliation using a shared electronic health care record. J Patient Saf 2011;7(3):147–53.
34. Nebeker JR, Hurdle JF, Bair BD. Future history: medical informatics in geriatrics. J Gerontol A Biol Sci Med Sci 2003;58(9):M820–M5.
35. Shabo A. Independent health record banks for older people—the ultimate integration of dispersed and disparate medical records. Inform Health Soc Care 2010;35(3–4): 188–99.
36. Demiris G, Doorenbos AZPRN, Towle C. Ethical considerations regarding the use of technology for older adults: the case of telehealth. Res Gerontol Nurs 2009;2(2): 128–36.
37. Wade V, Karnon J, Elshaug A, et al. A systematic review of economic analyses of telehealth services using real time video communication. BMC Health Serv Res 2010;10(1):233.
38. Paré G, Jaana M, Sicotte C. Systematic review of home telemonitoring for chronic diseases: the evidence base. J Am Med Informat Assoc 2007;14(3):269–77.
39. Hill RD, Luptak MK, Rupper RW, et al. Review of Veterans Health Administration telemedicine interventions. Am J Manag Care. 2010;16(12 Suppl HIT):e302–10.
40. Surescripts Available at: www.surescripts.com. Accessed September 13, 2011.
41. Surescripts Available at www.surescripts.com. Accessed September 12, 2011.
42. Bell DS, Friedman MA. E-prescribing and the Medicare Modernization Act of 2003. Health Affairs 2005;24(5):1159–69.
43. Weingart SN, Simchowitz B, Shiman L, et al. Clinicians' assessments of electronic medication safety alerts in ambulatory care. Arch Intern Med 2009; 169(17):1627–32.
44. Kuo GM, Phillips RL, Graham D, et al. Medication errors reported by US family physicians and their office staff. Quality Saf Health Care 2008;17(4):286–90.
45. Lapane KL, Waring ME, Dube C, et al. E-prescribing and patient safety: results from a mixed methods study. Amer J Pharm Ben, In press.
46. Lawrence D. Steps forward on e-prescribing. As e-prescribing becomes more widespread, even hospital organizations without full EMR implementation are seeing gains in clinician workflow and patient safety. Healthc Inform 2010;27(5):24–6.
47. Hor C, O'Donnell J, Murphy A, et al. General practitioners' attitudes and preparedness towards Clinical Decision Support in e-Prescribing (CDS-eP) adoption in the West of Ireland: a cross sectional study. BMC Med Inform Decision Making 2010; 10(1):2.
48. Devine EB, Hollingworth W, Hansen RN, et al. Electronic prescribing at the point of care: a time-motion study in the primary care setting. Health Serv Res 2010;45(1): 152–71.
49. Lapane KL, Rosen RK, Dube C. Perceptions of e-prescribing efficiencies and inefficiencies in ambulatory care. Int J Med Inform 2011;80(1):39–46.
50. Goldman RE, Dube C, Lapane KL. Beyond the basics: refills by electronic prescribing. Int J Med Inform 2010;79(7):507–14.
51. Ammenwerth E, Schnell-Inderst P, Machan C, et al. The effect of electronic prescribing on medication errors and adverse drug events: a systematic review. J Am Med Inform Assoc 2008;15(5):585–600.
52. Garg AX, Adhikari NKJ, McDonald H, et al. Effects of Computerized clinical decision support systems on practitioner performance and patient outcomes. JAMA 2005; 293(10):1223–38.
53. Devine EB, Hansen RN, Wilson-Norton JL, et al. The impact of computerized provider order entry on medication errors in a multispecialty group practice. J Am Med Inform Assoc 2010;17(1):78–84.

54. Teich JM, Osheroff JA, Pifer EA, et al. Clinical decision support in electronic prescribing: recommendations and an action plan. J Am Med Inform Assoc 2005; 12(4):365–76.

55. Durieux P, Trinquart L, Colombet I, et al. Computerized advice on drug dosage to improve prescribing practice. Cochrane Database Syst Rev 2008;3:CD002894.

56. Jaspers MWM, Smeulers M, Vermeulen H, et al. Effects of clinical decision-support systems on practitioner performance and patient outcomes: a synthesis of high-quality systematic review findings. J Am Med Inform Assoc 2011;18(3):327–34.

57. Hemens B, Holbrook A, Tonkin M, et al. Computerized clinical decision support systems for drug prescribing and management: a decision-maker-researcher partnership systematic review. Implement Sci 2011;6(1):89.

58. Shojania KG, Jennings A, Mayhew A, et al. The effects of on-screen, point of care computer reminders on processes and outcomes of care. Cochrane Database of Systematic Reviews. 2010;3.

59. Bryan C, Boren SA. The use and effectiveness of electronic clinical decision support tools in the ambulatory/primary care setting: a systematic review of the literature. Inform Prim Care 2008;16(2):79–91.

60. Figge HL. Electronic prescribing in the ambulatory care setting. Am J Health Syst Pharm 2009;66(1):16–8.

61. Tamblyn R, Huang A, Perreault R, et al. The medical office of the 21st century (MOXXI): effectiveness of computerized decision-making support in reducing inappropriate prescribing in primary care. CMAJ 2003;169(6):549–56.

62. Raebel MA, Charles J, Dugan J, et al. Randomized Trial to improve prescribing safety in ambulatory elderly patients. J Am Geriatr Soc 2007;55(7):977–85.

63. Weber V, White A, McIlvried R. An electronic medical record (EMR)-based intervention to reduce polypharmacy and falls in an ambulatory rural elderly population. J Gen Int Med 2008;23(4):399–404.

64. Smith DH, Perrin N, Feldstein A, et al. The impact of prescribing safety alerts for elderly persons in an electronic medical record: an interrupted time series evaluation. Arch Intern Med 2006;166(10):1098–104.

65. Simon SR, Smith DH, Feldstein AC, et al. Computerized prescribing alerts and group academic detailing to reduce the use of potentially inappropriate medications in older people. J Am Geriatr Soc 2006;54(6):963–8.

66. Monane M, Matthias DM, Nagle BA, et al. Improving prescribing patterns for the elderly through an online drug utilization review intervention: a system linking the physician, pharmacist, and computer. JAMA 1998;280(14):1249–52.

67. Cunningham TR, Geller ES, Clarke SW. Impact of electronic prescribing in a hospital setting: a process-focused evaluation. International Journal of Medical Informatics. 2008 Aug;77(8):546–54.

68. Terrell KM, Perkins AJ, Dexter PR, et al. Computerized decision support to reduce potentially inappropriate prescribing to older emergency department patients: a randomized, controlled trial. J Am Geriatr Soc 2009;57(8):1388–94.

69. Peterson JF, Kuperman GJ, Shek C, et al. Guided prescription of psychotropic medications for geriatric inpatients. Arch Intern Med 2005;165(7):802–7.

70. Agostini JV, Zhang Y, Inouye SK. Use of a computer-based reminder to improve sedative–hypnotic prescribing in older hospitalized patients. J Am Geriatr Soc 2007;55(1):43–8.

71. Mattison MLP, Afonso KA, Ngo LH, et al. Preventing potentially inappropriate medication use in hospitalized older patients with a computerized provider order entry warning system. Arch Intern Med 2010;170(15):1331–6.

72. Colón-Emeric CS, Schmader KE, Twersky J, et al. Development and pilot testing of computerized order entry algorithms for geriatric problems in nursing homes. J Am Geriatr Soc 2009;57(9):1644–53.
73. Yu P, Qiu Y, Crookes P. Computer-based nursing documentation in nursing homes: A feasibility study. Studies Health Tech Informat 2006;122:570–4.
74. Brandeis GH, Hogan M, Murphy M, et al. Electronic health record implementation in community nursing homes. J Am Med Dir Assoc 2007;8(1):31–4.
75. Vogelsmeier AA, Halbesleben JRB, Scott-Cawiezell JR. Technology implementation and workarounds in the nursing home. J Am Med Inform Assoc 2008;15(1):114–9.
76. Pierson S, Hansen R, Greene S, et al. Preventing medication errors in long-term care: results and evaluation of a large scale web-based error reporting system. Qual Saf Health Care 2007;16(4):297–302.
77. Gurwitz JH, Field TS, Rochon P, et al. Effect of computerized provider order entry with clinical decision support on adverse drug events in the long-term care setting. J Am Geriatr Soc 2008;56(12):2225–33.
78. Field TS, Rochon P, Lee M, et al. Computerized clinical decision support during medication ordering for long-term care residents with renal insufficiency. J Am Med Inform Assoc 2009;16(4):480–5.
79. Judge J, Field TS, DeFlorio M, et al. Prescribers' responses to alerts during medication ordering in the long term care setting. J Am Med Inform Assoc 2006; 13(4):385–90.
80. Lapane KL, Hughes CM, Daiello LA, et al. Effect of a pharmacist-led multicomponent intervention focusing on the medication monitoring phase to prevent potential adverse drug events in nursing homes. J Am Geriatr Soc 2011;59(7):1238–45.
81. Lapane KL, Hughes CM, Christian JB, et al. Evaluation of the Fleetwood model of long-term care pharmacy. J Am Med Dir Assoc 2011;12(5):355–63.
82. Ward R, Stevens C, Brentnall P, et al. The attitudes of health care staff to information technology: a comprehensive review of the research literature. Health Info Libr J 2008;25(2):81–97.
83. Barber N, Cornford T, Klecun E. Qualitative evaluation of an electronic prescribing and administration system. Qual Saf Health Care 2007;16(4):271–8.
84. Desroches CM, Agarwal R, Angst CM, et al. Differences between integrated and stand-alone E-prescribing systems have implications for future use. Health Aff (Millwood). 2010;29(12):2268–77.
85. Abdel-Qader DH, Cantrill JA, Tully MP. Satisfaction predictors and attitudes towards electronic prescribing systems in three UK hospitals. Pharm World Sci 2010;32(5):581–93.
86. Hellstrom L, Waern K, Montelius E, et al. Physicians' attitudes towards ePrescribing—evaluation of a Swedish full-scale implementation. BMC Med Inform Decis Mak 2009;9:37.
87. Ash JS, Sittig DF, Dykstra R, et al. The unintended consequences of computerized provider order entry: findings from a mixed methods exploration. Int J Med Inform 2009;78(Suppl 1):S69–S76.
88. AHRQ. Findings from the Evaluation of E-Prescribing Pilot Sites. 2007; Publication no. 07-0047-EF Available at: http://norc.uchicago.edu/NR/rdonlyres/5DBBB0A9-5EFF-404E-9BA5-40009373A6E1/0/FindingsFromTheEvaluationofEPrescribing PilotSites_200704.pdf. Accessed August 17, 2011.
89. Smith AD. Barriers to accepting e-prescribing in the USA. J Health Care Qual Assur 2006;19(2):158–80.
90. Redwood S, Rajakumar A, Hodson J, et al. Does the implementation of an electronic prescribing system create unintended medication errors? A study of the sociotechnical context through the analysis of reported medication incidents. BMC Med Inform Decis Mak 2011 May;11.

91. Committee on Data Standards for Patient Safety. Key capabilities of an electronic heatlh record system. Washington, DC: Institute of Medicine National Academies Press; 2003.

92. Poon E, Jha A, Christino M, et al. Assessing the level of healthcare information technology adoption in the United States: a snapshot. BMC Med Inform Decis Mak 2006;6(1):1.

93. Ferris. N. Long-term care lags in health IT. Government health IT: A guide to public policy and its applications in health IT. Available at: http://govhealthitcom/article90387-08-24-05-Web. 2005. Accessed September 13, 2011.

94. Alexander GL, Wakefield DS. Information technology sophistication in nursing homes. J Am Med Dir Assoc 2009;10(6):398–407.

95. Rantz MJPRNF, Skubic M, Alexander G, et al. Developing a comprehensive electronic health record to enhance nursing care coordination, use of technology, and research. J Gerontol Nurs 2010;36(1):13–7.

96. Microsoft Server Product Portfolio. Available at: http://www.css-security.com/wp-content/downloads/papers/hcrmanorcare.pdf. Accessed September 25, 2011.

97. Lapane KL, Waring ME, Schneider KL, et al. A mixed method study of the merits of E-prescribing drug alerts in primary care. J Gen Intern Med 2008;23(4):442–6.

98. Phansalkar S, Edworthy J, Hellier E, et al. A review of human factors principles for the design and implementation of medication safety alerts in clinical information systems. J Am Med Inform Assoc 2010;17(5):493–501.

99. van der Sijs H, Aarts J, Vulto A,et al. Overriding of drug safety alerts in computerized physician order entry. J Am Med Inform Assoc 2006;13(2):138–47.

100. Moxey A, Robertson J, Newby D, et al. Computerized clinical decision support for prescribing: provision does not guarantee uptake. J Am Med Inform Assoc 2010; 17(1):25–33.

101. Hume AL, Quilliam BJ, Goldman R, et al. Alternatives to potentially inappropriate medications for use in e-prescribing software: triggers and treatment algorithms. BMJ Qual Saf 2011.

102. Hammar T, Nyström S, Petersson G, et al. Patients satisfied with e-prescribing in Sweden: a survey of a nationwide implementation. J Pharm Health Serv Res 2011;2(2):97–105.

103. Lapane KL, Dube C, Schneider KL, et al. Patient perceptions regarding electronic prescriptions: Is the geriatric patient ready? J Am Geriatr Soc 2007;55(8):1254–9.

104. Kaur S, Mitchell G, Vitetta L, et al. Interventions that can reduce inappropriate prescribing in the elderly: a systematic review. Drugs Aging 2009;26(12):1013–28.

105. Loganathan M, Singh S, Franklin BD, et al. Interventions to optimise prescribing in care homes: systematic review. Age Ageing 2011;40(2):150–62.

106. Yourman L, Concato J, Agostini JV. Use of computer decision support interventions to improve medication prescribing in older adults: a systematic review. Am J Geriatr Pharmacother 2008;6(2):119–29.

Tools to Reduce Polypharmacy

Murthy Gokula, MD[a],*, Holly M. Holmes, MD[b]

KEYWORDS

- Inappropriate medication • Medication management
- Elderly • Polypharmacy

Approximately one-third of drugs prescribed in the United States may be unnecessary.[1] Older adults use higher numbers of medications compared with younger age groups, primarily because of increased numbers of comorbid conditions and greater numbers of physicians involved in their care, putting them at higher risk of polypharmacy. The use of multiple medications increases the risk for adverse drug events and adverse health outcomes.[2,3] Medication management is of utmost significance in older adults because of changes in body composition, physical function, social environment, and limiting finances with increasing age. Adding or stopping a medication in an older person should focus on improving function or quality of life, a core principle in the management of chronic illnesses in the elderly (**Box 1**).

Older adults are the largest consumers of prescription medications, and over-the-counter (OTC) medications and dietary supplements among older adults are on the rise in the United States. Qato and colleagues[4] conducted a survey in 3500 community-dwelling older adults and found that 29% took 5 or more prescription medications, 42% took at least 1 or more OTC medications, and 49% took at least 1 or more dietary supplements. Approximately 50 new medications enter the market each year, and the use of prescription drugs will continue to increase. Direct-to-consumer marketing and the continued focus on life-saving and life-sustaining therapies increases the reliance on medication therapy in older adults.

Adverse drug reactions (ADRs) are likely with excessive medication use; the risk of an ADR increases with increased medication number.[5] ADRs may be caused by drug-drug or drug-disease interactions and by the use of medications considered inappropriate in the elderly, and ADRs are a major cause of costly hospitalization in

The authors have no relevant financial disclosures to report in relationship to this manuscript. Dr Holmes is supported by grant K23AG038476 from the National Institute on Aging.

[a] Geriatric Medicine Fellowship Program, St. Luke's Hospital/University of Toledo, 6005 Monclova Road, Suite 220, Maumee, OH 43537, USA
[b] Department of General Internal Medicine, University of Texas MD Anderson Cancer Center, 1400 Pressler, Unit 1465, Houston, TX 77030, USA
* Corresponding author.
E-mail address: murthy.gokula@utoledo.edu

Box 1
Definitions

Polypharmacy is defined as the use of multiple medications or duplicative medications that cause increased risk for drug-drug and drug-disease interactions.

Polymedicine or **polytherapy** describes the use of multiple medications prescribed appropriately for treating multiple comorbid conditions.

The prescribing cascade refers to the use of a medication that results in an adverse drug event that is mistaken for a new diagnosis and treated with another medication, thus, increasing the risk for further adverse drug events.

---

older adults.[5,6] Decreasing medication number and, specifically, decreasing the use of inappropriate medications, may reduce the risk of an ADR.

INTERVENTIONS TO IMPROVE PRESCRIBING

A systematic review by Loganathan and coworkers[7] summarized the effect of interventions to improve prescribing and concluded that staff education in the form of academic detailing has strong evidence for improvement in prescribing in nursing homes and care homes. The successful studies in the review included interactive techniques: (1) academic detailing with face-to-face interaction between a group of experts and prescribing physicians, (2) nursing workshops, and (3) family education. In this review, the use of computerized clinical decision support systems improved appropriate prescribing, and multidisciplinary team meetings including communication among health care professionals increased appropriate prescribing. Pharmacist medication reviews to improve appropriate prescribing were significantly successful in only 1 study.[7] In the United States, a monthly pharmacist medication review is mandatory in long-term care. A systematic review found mixed results for different approaches used to improve appropriate prescribing. However, because of the heterogeneity of study interventions and measures of suboptimal prescribing used in the studies, clear conclusions regarding the most effective interventions were not reached.[8]

Multidisciplinary case conferences involving a geriatrician have been shown to be effective interventions to improve prescribing in both community and hospital settings.[9] It is not clear whether combined strategies undertaken simultaneously have a synergistic effect, but a combination of intervention strategies is likely required to reduce polypharmacy. These combinations could include educational intervention, regular medication review, geriatrics consultation, multidisciplinary team meetings, computerized decision support systems, regulatory policies and procedures, interventions to improve documentation regarding medication indication, and increased vigilance during transitions in care.[9]

Although all of the above strategies may not be routinely available for the busy practicing clinician, a number of tools have been created to aid in medication management. These tools have been developed in various settings and have varying levels of support for their use. Ultimately, to reduce harmful polypharmacy and in settings in which combined interventions are not in use, evidence-based tools need to be incorporated into regular practice to aid in optimizing an older patient's medication regimen. We review a number of such tools that address polypharmacy in the context of their supporting evidence.

THE BEERS CRITERIA

This explicit list of medications (**Tables 1** and **2**) was created by expert consensus in 1991 and originally intended to identify inappropriate medication use in nursing home residents.[10] In 1997, the criteria were revised to apply more generally to persons 65 and older.[11] The criteria were again updated in 2003 with a list of 48 inappropriate medications or drug classes and a list of 20 combinations of medications inappropriate in the setting of specific diagnoses and conditions.[12] The Beers criteria have been updated recently to incorporate the most current evidence according to expert consensus and will be published with the support of the American Geriatrics Society in 2012.

The Beers criteria have been widely adopted in the United States and elsewhere and have been studied in numerous settings.[13] The disadvantages of the criteria are that many of the drugs are older and out of use, and there is insufficient evidence to include some drugs on the list. Further, the harm resulting from the use of some of the inappropriate medications on the list may be minor compared with other inappropriate prescribing, such as under- or overuse of medications, drug-drug interactions, drug-disease interactions, or drug duplication.[14] Finally, the Beers criteria are consensus based, and the reliability of the Delphi process to generate such a list is not definitively established.[15]

Ultimately, the Beers list may be most attractive because it is easy to use, both in clinical and research settings, because lists of drugs to avoid require little individualization or time-consuming decision-making during a busy clinic visit. The list can be easily incorporated into computerized decision support systems to prevent inappropriate use and in reviews of administrative claims databases to determine the prevalence and predictors of use.

IMPROVED PRESCRIBING IN THE ELDERLY TOOL, ALSO KNOWN AS THE CANADIAN CRITERIA

The Improved Prescribing in the Elderly Tool (IPET)[16] was developed by applying criteria for inappropriate medications from McLeod and colleagues[17] to 362 inpatients, resulting in 45 different medications in 14 classes of drugs considered inappropriate. Although the IPET is similar to the Beers criteria, the Beers list identifies more medications that are potentially inappropriate.[18] There is insufficient convincing evidence regarding the use of IPET to reduce the incidence of adverse drug events, health resource utilization, or mortality.[19]

SCREENING TOOL TO ALERT DOCTORS TO RIGHT TREATMENTS AND SCREENING TOOL OF OLDER PERSONS' POTENTIALLY INAPPROPRIATE PRESCRIPTIONS

These tools[20,21] were developed by an interdisciplinary team of geriatricians, primary care physicians, pharmacists, geriatric psychiatrists, and pharmacologists in Ireland. The Screening Tool to Alert Doctors to Right Treatments (START) tool consists of 22 evidence-based indicators of drugs commonly omitted by physicians. START is validated, with a high interrater reliability between physicians and pharmacists.[22] The Screening Tool of Older Persons' Potentially Inappropriate Prescriptions (STOPP) includes 65 indicators, mostly focused on drug-drug and drug-disease interactions that influence the risk for falls and duplications of common medication classes. The items are grouped based on human physiologic systems and by drug class. A randomized, controlled trial using START and STOPP in combination with the Medication Appropriateness Index (MAI) and Assessment of Underutilization index to test appropriate prescribing at hospital discharge and 6 months later

Table 1

2002 Criteria for potentially inappropriate medication use in older adults: independent of diagnoses or conditions

Drug	Concern	Severity Rating (High or Low)
Propoxyphene (Darvon) and combination products (Darvon with ASA, Darvon-N, and Darvocet-N)	Offers few analgesic advantages over acetaminophen, yet has the adverse effects of other narcotic drugs.	Low
Indomethacin (Indocin and Indocin SR)	Of all available nonsteroidal anti-inflammatory drugs, this drug produces the most CNS adverse effects.	High
Pentazocine (Talwin)	Narcotic analgesic that causes more CNS adverse effects, including confusion and hallucinations, more commonly than other narcotic drugs. Additionally, it is a mixed agonist and antagonist.	High
Trimethobenzamide (Tigan)	One of the least effective antiemetic drugs, yet it can cause extrapyramidal adverse effects.	High
Muscle relaxants and antispasmodics: methocarbamol (Robaxin), carisoprodol (Soma), chlorzoxazone (Paraflex), metaxalone (Skelaxin), cyclobenzaprine (Flexeril), and oxybutynin (Ditropan). Do not consider the extended-release Ditropan XL	Most muscle relaxants and antispasmodic drugs are poorly tolerated by elderly patients, since these cause anticholinergic adverse effects, sedation, and weakness. Additionally, their effectiveness at doses tolerated by elderly patients is questionable.	High
Flurazepam (Dalmane)	This benzodiazepine hypnotic has an extremely long half-life in elderly patients (often days), producing prolonged sedation and increasing the incidence of falls and fracture. Medium- or short-acting benzodiazepines are preferable.	High
Amitriptyline (Elavil), chlordiazepoxide-amitriptyline (Limbitrol), and perphenazine-amitriptyline (Triavil)	Because of its strong anticholinergic and sedation properties, amitriptyline is rarely the antidepressant of choice for elderly patients.	High
Doxepin (Sinequan)	Because of its strong anticholinergic and sedation properties, doxepin is rarely the antidepressant of choice for elderly patients.	High
Meprobamate (Miltown and Equanil)	This is a highly addictive and sedating anxiolytic. Those using meprobamate for prolonged periods may become addicted and may need to be withdrawn slowly.	High

(continued on next page)

Table 1
(continued)

Drug	Concern	Severity Rating (High or Low)
Doses of short-acting benzodiazepines: doses greater than lorazepam (Ativan), 3 mg; oxazepam (Serax), 60 mg; alprazolam (Xanax), 2 mg; temazepam (Restoril), 15 mg; and triazolam (Halcion), 0.25 mg	Because of increased sensitivity to benzoadiazepines in elderly patients, smaller doses may be effective as well as safer. Total daily doses should rarely exceed the suggested maximums.	High
Long-acting benzodiazepines: chlordiazepoxide (Librium), chlordiazepoxide-amitriptyline (Limbitrol), clidinium-chlordiazepoxide (Librax), diazepam (Valium), quazepam (Doral), halazepam (Paxipam), and chlorazepate (Tranxene)	These drugs have a long half-life in elderly patients (often several days), producing prolonged sedation and increasing the risk of falls and fractures. Short- and intermediate-acting benzodiazepines are preferred if a benzodiazepine is required.	High
Disopyramide (Norpace and Norpace CR)	Of all antiarrhythmic drugs, this is the most potent negative inotrope and therefore may induce heart failure in elderly patients. It is also strongly anticholinergic. Other antiarrhythmic drugs should be used.	High
Digoxin (Lanoxin) (should not exceed >0.125 mg/d except when treating atrial arrhythmias)	Decreased renal clearance may lead to increased risk of toxic effects.	Low
Short-acting dipyridamole (Persantine). Do not consider the long-acting dipyridamole (which has better properties than the short-acting in older adults) with the patients with artificial heart valves	May cause orthostatic hypotension.	Low
Methyldopa (Aldomet) and methyldopa-hydrochlorothiazide (Aldoril)	May cause bradycardia and exacerbate depression in elderly patients.	High
Reserpine at doses >0.25 mg	May induce depression, impotence, sedation, and orthostatic hypotension.	Low
Chlorpropamide (Diabinese)	It has a prolonged half-life in elderly patients and could cause prolonged hypoglycemia. Additionally, it is the only oral hypoglycemic agent that causes SIADH.	High

(continued on next page)

Table 1
(continued)

Drug	Concern	Severity Rating (High or Low)
Gastrointestinal antispasmodic drugs: dicyclomine (Bentyl), hyoscyamine (Levsin and Levsinex), propantheline (Pro-Banthine), belladonna alkaloids (Donnafal and others, and clidinium-chlordiazepoxide (Librax)	GI antispasmodic drugs are highly anticholinergic and have uncertain effectiveness, These drugs should be avoided (especially for long-term use).	High
Anticholinergics and antihistamines: chlorpheniramine (Chlor-Trimenton), diphenhydramine (Benadryl), hydroxyzine (Vistaril and Atarax), cyproheptadine (Periactin), promethazine (Phenergan), tripelennamine, dexchlorpheniramine (Polaramine)	All nonprescription and many prescription antihistamines may have potent anticholinergic properties. Nonanticholinergic antihistamines are preferred in elderly patients when treating allergic reactions.	High
Diphenhydramine (Benadryl)	May cause confusion and sedation. Should not be used as a hypnotic, and when used to treat emergency allergic reactions, it should be used in the smallest possible dose.	High
Ergot mesyloids (Hydergine), and cyclandelate (Cyclospasmol)	Have not been shown to be effective in the doses studied.	Low
Ferrous sulfate >325 mg/d	Doses >325 mg/d do not dramatically increase the amount absorbed but greatly increase the incidence of constipation.	Low
All barbiturates (except Phenobarbital) except when used to control seizures	Are highly addictive and cause more adverse effects than most sedative or hypnotic drugs in elderly patients.	High
Meperidine (Demerol)	Not an effective oral analgesic in doses commonly used. May cause confusion and has many disadvantages to other narcotic drugs.	High
Ticlopidine (Ticlid)	Has been shown to be no better than aspirin in preventing clotting and may be considerably more toxic. Safer, more effective alternatives exist.	High
Ketorolac (Toradol)	Immediate and long-term use should be avoided in older persons, since a significant number have asymptomatic GI pathologic conditions.	High

(continued on next page)

Table 1 (continued)		
Drug	Concern	Severity Rating (High or Low)
Amphetamines and anorexic agents	These drugs have potential for causing dependence, hypertension, angina, and myocardial infarction.	High
Long-term use of full-dosage, longer half-life, non–COX-selective NSAIDS: naproxen (Naprosyn, Avaprox, and Aleve), oxaprozin (Daypro), and piroxicam (Feldene)	Have the potential to produce GI bleeding, renal failure, high blood pressure, and heart failure.	High
Daily fluoxetine (Prozac)	Long half-life of drug and risk of producing excessive CNS stimulation, sleep disturbances, and increasing agitation. Safer alternatives exist.	High
Long-term use of stimulant laxatives: bisacodyl (Dulcolax), cascara sagrada, and Neoloid except in the presence of opiate analgesic use	May exacerbate bowel dysfunction.	High
Amiodarone (Cordarone)	Associated with QT interval problems and risk of provoking torsades de pointes. Lack of efficacy in older adults.	High
Orphenadrinie (Norflex)	Causes more sedation and anticholinergic adverse effects than safer alternatives.	High
Guanethidine (Ismelin)	May cause orthostatic hypotension. Safer alternatives exist.	High
Guanadrel (hylorel)	May cause orthostatic hypotension.	High
Cyclandelate (Cyclospasmol)	Lack of efficacy.	Low
Isoxsurpine (Vasodilan)	Lack of efficacy.	Low
Nitrofurantoin (Macrodantin)	Potential for renal impairment. Safer alternative available.	High
Doxazosin (Cardura)	Potential for hypotension, dry mouth, and urinary problems.	Low
Methyltestosterone (Android, Virilon, and Testrad)	Potential for prostatic hypertrophy and cardiac problems.	High
Thioridazine (Mellaril)	Greater potential for CNS and extrapyramidal adverse effects.	High
Mesoridazine (Serentil)	CNS and extrapyramidal adverse effects.	High
Short-acting nifedipine (Procardia and Adalat)	Potential for hypotension and constipation.	High
Clonidine (Catapres)	Potential for orthostatic hypotension and CNS adverse effects.	Low

(continued on next page)

Table 1
(continued)

Drug	Concern	Severity Rating (High or Low)
Mineral oil	Potential for aspiration and adverse effects. Safer alternatives available.	High
Cimetidine (Tagamet)	CNS adverse effects including confusion.	Low
Ethacrynic acid (Edecrin)	Potential for hypertension and fluid imbalances. Safer alternative available.	Low
Desiccated thyroid	Concerns about cardiac effects. Safer alternative available.	High
Amphetamines (excluding methylphenidate hydrochloride and anorexics)	CNS stimulant adverse effects.	High
Estrogens only (oral)	Evidence of the carcinogenic (breast and endometrial cancer) potential of these agents and lack of cardioprotective effect in older women.	Low

Abbreviations: CNS, central nervous system; COX, cyclooxygenase; GI, gastrointestinal; NSAIDs, nonsteroidal anti-inflammatory drugs; SIADH, syndrome of inappropriate antidiuretic hormone secretion.

From Fick DM, Cooper JW, Wade WE, et al. Updating the Beers criteria for potentially inappropriate medication use in older adults: results of a US consensus panel of experts. Arch Intern Med 2003;163(22):2716–24; with permission.

showed that the use of these criteria, in combination, showed lower rates of polypharmacy, higher rates of correct drug dosing, and reduced drug-drug interactions. The effects were sustained 6 months after discharge.[23] A comparative study of STOPP and the Beers criteria to detect inappropriate prescribing showed the higher sensitivity of the STOPP criteria.[24] The advantages of START and STOPP criteria are (1) good interrater reliability, (2) inclusion of medications used both in the United States and in Europe, (3) logical organization and structure with easy-to-use explicit lists of medication criteria, and (4) short time to complete, usually about 3 minutes.

MEDICATION APPROPRIATENESS INDEX

The MAI uses implicit criteria to measure elements of appropriate prescribing (**Table 3**). It consists of 10 elements considered necessary for appropriate prescribing, including indication, effectiveness, appropriate dose, practical and correct directions, absence of interactions, lack of therapeutic duplication, appropriate duration, and low cost.[25] The MAI involves the use of clinical judgment to assess each criterion, but has operational definitions and explicit instructions to standardize the rating process. The ratings are scored, with different weights for some of the elements considered more important.[26] Of the 10 components in the MAI, 3 (indication, effectiveness, and duplication) can be used without the other 7 to detect polypharmacy and inappropriate prescribing.[27] The main advantages of the MAI are that it can be used in

Table 2
2002 Criteria for potentially inappropriate medication use in older adults: considering diagnoses or conditions

Disease or Condition	Drug	Concern	Severity Rating (High or Low)
Heart failure	Disopyramide (Norpace), and high sodium content drugs (sodium and sodium salts [alginate bicarbonate, biphosphate, citrate, phosphate, salicylate, and sulfate])	Negative inotropic effect. Potential to promote fluid retention and exacerbation of heart failure.	High
Hypertension	Phenylpropanolamine hydrochloride (removed from the market in 2001), pseudoephedrine: diet pills and amphetamines	May produce elevation of blood pressure secondary to sympathomimetic activity.	High
Gastric or duodenal ulcers	NSAIDS and aspirin (>325 mg) (coxibs excluded)	May exacerbate existing ulcers or produce new/additional ulcers.	High
Seizures or epilepsy	Clozapine (Clozaril), chlorpromazine (Thorazine), thioridazine (Mellaril), and thiothixene (Navane)	May lower seizure thresholds.	High
Blood clotting disorders or receiving anticoagulant therapy	Aspirin, NSAIDs, dipyridamole (Persantin), ticlopidine (Ticlid), and clopidogrel (Plavix)	May prolong clotting time and elevate INR values or inhibit platelet aggregation, resulting in an increased potential for bleeding.	High
Bladder outflow obstruction	Anticholinergics and antihistamines, gastrointestinal antispasmodics, muscle relaxants, oxybutynin (Ditropan), flavoxate (Urispas), anticholinergics, antidepressants, decongestants, and tolterodine (Detrol)	May decrease urinary flow, leading to urinary retention.	High
Stress incontinence	α-Blockers (Doxazosin, Prazosin, and Terazosin), anticholinergics, tricyclic antidepressants (imipramine hydrochloride, doxepin hydrochloride, and amitriptyline hydrochloride), and long-acting benzodiazepines	My produce polyruia and worsening of incontinence.	High

(continued on next page)

Table 2
(continued)

Disease or Condition	Drug	Concern	Severity Rating (High or Low)
Arrhythmias	Tricyclic antidepressants (imipramine hydrochloride)	Concern due to proarrhythmic effects and ability to produce QT interval changes.	High
Insomnia	Decongestants, theophylline (Theodur), methylphenidate (Ritalin), MAOIs, and amphetamines	Concern due to CNS stimulant effects.	High
Parkinson disease	Metoclopramide (Reglan), conventional antipsychotics, and tacrine (Cognex)	Concern due to their antidopaminergic/cholinergic effects.	High
Cognitive impairment	Barbiturates, anticholinergics, antispasmodics, and muscle relaxants. CNS stimulants: dextroAmphetamine (Adderall), methylphenidate (Rialin), methamphetamine (Desoxyn), and pemolin	Concern due to CNS-altering effects.	High
Depression	Long-term benzodiazepine use. Sympatholytic agents: methyldopa (Aldomet), reserpine, and guanethidine (Ismelin)	May produce or exacerbate depression.	High
Anorexia and malnutrition	CNS stimulants: DextroAmphetamine (Adderall), methylphenidate (Ritalin), methamphetamine (Desoxyn), permolin, and fluoxetine (Prozac)	Concern due to appetite-suppressing effects.	High
Syncope or falls	Short- to intermediate-acting benzodiazepine and tricyclic antidepressants (imipramine hydrochooride, doxepin hydrochloride, and amitriptyline hydrochloride)	May produce ataxia, imipaired psychomotor function, syncope, and additional falls.	High
SIADH/ hyponatremia	SSRIs: fluoxetine (Prozac), citalopram (Celexa), fluvoxamine (Luvox), paroxetine (Paxil), and sertraline (Zoloft)	May exacerbate or cause SIADH.	Low
Seizure disorder	Bupropion (Wellbutrin)	May lower seizure threshold.	High
Obesity	Olanzapine (Zyprexa)	May stimulate appetite and increase weight gain.	Low

(continued on next page)

Disease or Condition	Drug	Concern	Severity Rating (High or Low)
Table 2 *(continued)*			
COPD	Long-acting benzodiazepines: chlordiazepoxide (Librium), chlordiazepoxide-amitriptylinie (Limbitrol), clidinium-chlordiazepoxide (Librax), diazepam (Valium), quazepam (Doral), halazepam (Pasipam), and chlorazepate (Tranxene). β-blockers: propranolol	CNS adverse effects. May induce respiratory depression. May exacerbate or cause respiratory depression.	High
Chronic constipation	Calcium channel blockers, anticholinergics, and tricyclic antidepressant (imipramine hydrochloride, doxepin hydrochloride, and amitriptyline hydrochloride)	May exacerbate constipation.	Low

Abbreviations: CNS, central nervous system; COPD, chronie obstructive pulmonary disease; INR, international normalized ratio; MAOIs, monoamine oxidase inhibitors; NSAIDs, nonsteroidal anti-inflammatory drugs; SIADH, syndrome of inappropriate antidiuretic hormone secretion; SSRIs, selective serotonin reuptake inhibitors.

From Fick DM, Cooper JW, Wade WE, et al. Updating the Beers criteria for potentially inappropriate medication use in older adults: results of a US consensus panel of experts. Arch Intern Med 2003;163(22):2716–24; with permission.

inpatient and ambulatory settings, has excellent intra- and interrater reliability, and has face and content validity. The main disadvantages are that it takes at least 10 minutes to complete the entire tool, and it does not address the underuse of appropriate prescribing, like the START tool, for example. The MAI has been linked to adverse outcomes in smaller studies[28] but has not been extensively used in various larger settings.

FIT FOR THE AGED CRITERIA

In this scheme, medications are graded based on Fit for the Aged Criteria (FORTA) class[29]: A, indispensible, with obvious benefit; B, proven efficacy but limited effects or possible safety concerns; C, questionable efficacy or safety; and D, avoid. In a small pilot study in Germany,[30] patients admitted to a geriatric medical ward had medications assessed on admission and at discharge using the criteria, and changes were made according to the criteria and also to reduce drug interactions. There was no significant decrease in the total number of prescribed drugs or in the number of negatively assessed drugs. There was a significant increase in positively assessed drugs as well as appropriate prescribing. These criteria, while presenting a promising approach to medication use in older persons, need further validation in controlled studies before widespread use.

Table 3 Medication appropriateness index	
Item	**Weight**
Is there an indication for the drug?	3
Is the medication effective for the condition?	3
Is the dosage correct?	2
Are the directions correct?	2
Are the directions practical?	1
Are there clinically significant drug-drug interactions?	2
Are there clinically significant drug-disease/condition interactions?	2
Is there unnecessary duplication with other drug(s)?	1
Is the duration of therapy acceptable?	1
Is this drug the least expensive alternative compared to others of equal utility?	1

Data from Hanlon JT, Schmader KE, Samsa GP, et al. A method for assessing drug therapy appropriateness. J Clin Epidemiol 1992;45(10):1045–51 and Samsa GP, Hanlon JT, Schmader KE, et al. A summated score for the medication appropriateness index: development and assessment of clinimetric properties including content validity. J Clin Epidemiol 1994;47(8):891–96.

THE ASSESS, REVIEW, MINIMIZE, OPTIMIZE, REASSESS

The Assess, Review, Minimize, Optimize, Reassess[31] tool (**Table 4**) is a functional and interactive evidence-based practice tool that is designed for use in nursing home residents. The tool takes into account patients' clinical profiles and functional status, including physiologic reserves. It can be used in patients (1) receiving 9 or more medications, (2) seen for initial assessment, (3) with falls or behavioral disturbance,

Table 4 The ARMOR tool		
A	Assess	• Beers criteria • β-blockers • Pain medications • Antidepressants • Antipsychotics • Other psychotropics • Vitamins and supplements
R	Review	• Drug–disease interactions • Drug–drug interactions • Adverse drug reactions
M	Minimize	• Number of medications according to functional status rather than evidence-based medicine
O	Optimize	• For renal/hepatic clearance, PT/PTT, β-blockers, pacemaker function, anticonvulsants, pain medications, and hypoglycemics; gradual dose reduction for antidepressants
R	Reassess	• Functional/cognitive status in 1 week and as needed • Clinical status and medication compliance

From Haque R. ARMOR: a tool to evaluate polypharmacy in elderly persons. Annals of Long-Term Care 2009;17(6):26–30; with permission. Available at: http://www.annalsoflongtermcare.com/content/armor-a-tool-evaluate-polypharmacy-elderly-persons. Accessed January 28, 2012.

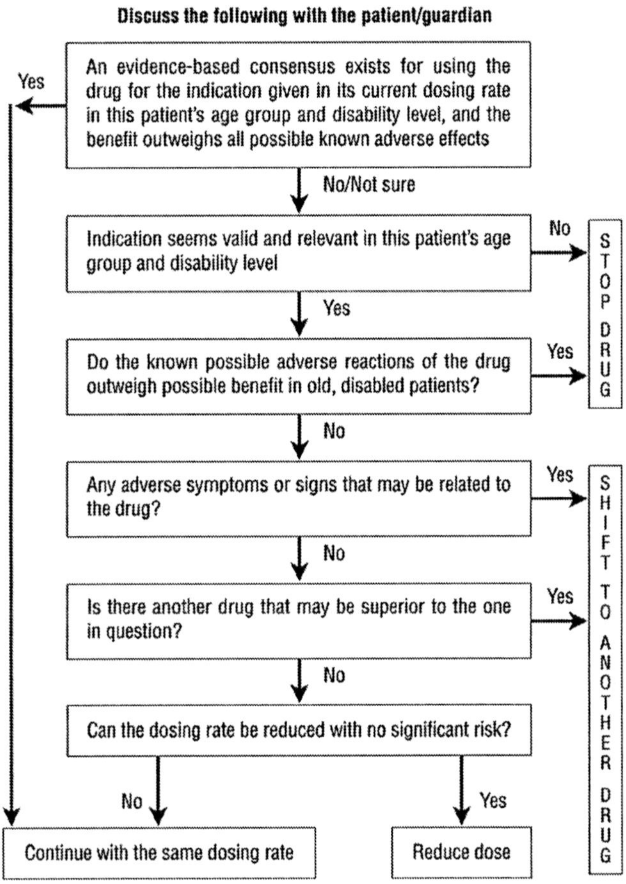

Discuss the following with the patient/guardian

Fig. 1. The Good Palliative-Geriatric Practice algorithm. (*From* Garfinkel D, Zur-Gil S, Ben-Israel J. The war against polypharmacy: a new cost-effective geriatric-palliative approach for improving drug therapy in disabled elderly people. Isr Med Assoc J 2007;9(6):430–34; with permission.)

and/or (4) admitted for rehabilitation. The primary goal of using this systematic approach is to improve functional status. It also incorporates making decisions on changing or discontinuing medications. The overall goal is to improve functional status and mobility, which are the main outcome measures for use of the tool. Its use has been shown to reduce polypharmacy, health care costs, and hospitalizations. However, it was only tested in one nursing facility.

GOOD PALLIATIVE-GERIATRIC PRACTICE ALGORITHM

The Good Palliative-Geriatric Practice algorithm[32] (**Fig. 1**) was a consensus-based flow chart developed in 2004 for nursing homes to reduce polypharmacy. The algorithm was used in 6 nursing homes in Israel, with 119 patients in the intervention group and 71 patients in the control group. There was a significant reduction in mortality, hospitalization, and cost. At the end of 1 year, an average of 2.8 drugs per patient was discontinued, and there were no significant adverse effects caused by

---

Box 2
Prescribing optimization method

1. Is the patient undertreated and is additional medication indicated?

2. Does the patient adhere to his/her medication schedule?

3. Which drug(s) can be withdrawn or which drug(s) is/are inappropriate for this patient?

4. Which adverse effects are present?

5. Which clinically relevant interactions are to be expected?

6. Should the dose frequency and/or form of the drug be adjusted?

Data from Drenth-van Maanen AC, van Marum RJ, Knol W, et al. Prescribing optimization method for improving prescribing in elderly patients receiving polypharmacy: results of application to case histories by general practitioners. Drugs Aging 2009;26(8):687–701.

---

discontinuation. The overall rate of drug discontinuation failure (that required resuming the original medication) was 18%, representing 10% of all the drugs. The 1-year mortality rate was 21% in the intervention group and 45% in the control group. Only 11.8% of the intervention group was readmitted to the hospital compared with 30% of the control group. There was a substantial decrease in the cost of drugs ($69 per patient) because of drug discontinuation.[33]

PATIENT-FOCUSED DRUG SURVEILLANCE

Patient-Focused Drug Surveillance[34] was an intervention study for elderly persons in nursing homes in Sweden. The intervention involved a physician-led, patient-focused approach, taking into account the patient's health condition to appropriately optimize medication therapy and reduce polypharmacy. Outcomes studied included mortality, health care utilization, number of medications, health status, and periodic evaluations of quality of drug treatment. The study found improvement in optimum prescribing, improved medication surveillance, and reduction in medication number. The advantage of this approach was the recognition of the need to discuss benefits and risks of drug therapy with frail older persons, accompanied by close monitoring and re-evaluation. The intervention was not described clearly enough to generate a quick reference tool, but the success of this type of intervention was the potential for a sustained change in practice.

GERIATRIC RISK ASSESSMENT MEDGUIDE

Geriatric Risk Assessment Medguide[35] is a clinical informatics tool that generates prospective monitoring plans based on potential risk for falls or for delirium within 24 hours of nursing home admission. Its use was evaluated in 25 nursing homes, assessing not only falls and delirium, but also hospitalizations owing to adverse drug events and mortality. The use of the Geriatric Risk Assessment Medguide tool significantly reduced the rate of delirium. The rates of hospitalization and mortality were lower but not statistically significant. The findings were lessened in residents with a longer length of stay.

PRESCRIBING OPTIMIZATION METHOD

The Prescribing Optimization Method[36] (**Box 2**) was developed to help general practitioners optimize medication use in older adults. POM is based on 6 questions that address the following: (1) undertreatment, (2) adherence, (3) drugs that can be discontinued or are inappropriate, (4) adverse drug events, (5) interactions, and (6) dosing frequency or formulation. Education of 45 primary care physicians about this approach resulted in improvement in optimum prescribing when applied to a patient case history. The advantage of its use in a clinical setting is that the 6 questions are open and allowed for clinical judgment and, after brief education, could promote better prescribing. Each question from the POM has a number of potential follow-up issues (eg, identification of drugs that are inappropriate) that individually could be time consuming.

ANTICHOLINERGIC RISK SCALE

To create the Anticholinergic Risk Scale (ARS),[37] (**Table 5**) the 500 most commonly prescribed drugs in the Veteran's Administration system were ranked according to anticholinergic potential and assigned a point value, and an individual's score was calculated by added the points for each drug. Increasing ARS score was significantly associated with anticholinergic adverse effects in a retrospective review of 132 geriatric patients and a prospective study of 117 primary care patients. Higher ARS scores have been associated with lower physical function scores[38] but not with mortality.[39] The advantages of the ARS score are the ease of calculating the score using a table given in the manuscript and the potential to reduce anticholinergic side effects; however, it could be time consuming and impractical in clinical settings compared with research settings.

Drug Burden Index

Similarly to the ARS, the drug burden index (DBI)[40] is a formula to describe anticholinergic and sedative burden. Total drug burden was calculated from a combination of data regarding anticholinergic properties, sedative effects, and total medication number, generating a single score for a patient. Applying the results to 3075 persons enrolled in the Health ABC study, increasing drug burden index was significantly correlated with functional and cognitive decline, although increasing medication number was not associated. Further studies have confirmed the association between increasing drug burden index and decreased physical and cognitive function.[41–45] Although the DBI could be incorporated readily into drug utilization review software, it may not be widely available, limiting its usability for most clinicians, unless they have access to a pharmacist or other consultant who may provide DBI scores. Further prospective intervention studies are needed to determine whether improving the DBI score results in better outcomes.

PRISCUS LIST

Developed in Germany, the PRISCUS list[46] is a consensus list of potentially inappropriate medications developed among experts in a process that included a qualitative analysis of inappropriate medication lists from multiple countries, a literature search for medications that cause adverse drug events, development of a preliminary list of inappropriate medications for use in Germany, and generation of the final PRISCUS list using a modified Delphi process. The final outcome was a list of 83 drugs that were rated as inappropriate for the elderly. The final list also contains recommendations for monitoring of laboratory values, dose adaptation, and therapeutic alternatives. The list was developed for use in Germany because of important differences in drugs approved on the market and in prescribing guidelines. Further prospective testing of the use of PRISCUS is needed.

Table 5
Anticholinergic risk scale[a]

3 Points	2 Points	1 Point
Amitriptyline hydrochloride	Amantadine hydrochloride	Carbidopa-levodopa
Atropine products	Baclofen	Entacapone
Benztropine mesylate	Cetirizine hydrochloride	Haloperidol
Carisoprodol	Cimetidine	Methocarbamol
Chlorpheniramine maleate	Clozapine	Metoclopramide hydrochloride
Chlorpromazine hydrochloride	Cyclobenzaprine hydrochloride	Mirtazapine
Dicyclomine hydrochloride	Loperamide hydrochloride	Paroxetine hydrochloride
Diphenhydramine hydrochloride	Loratadine	Pramipexole dihydrochloride
Fluphenazine hydrochloride	Nortriptyline hydrochloride	Quetiapine fumarate
Hydroxyzine hydrochloride and hydroxyzine pamoate	Olanzapine	Ranitidine hydrochloride
Hyoscyamine products	Prochlorperazine maleate	Risperidone
Imipramine hydrochloride	Pseudoephedrine hydrochloride–triprodlidine hydrochloride	Selegiline hydrochloride
Meclizine hydrochloride	Tolterodine tartrate	Trazodone hydrochloride
Oxybutynin chloride		Ziprasidone hydrochloride
Perphenazine		
Promethazine hydrochloride		
Thioridazine hydrochloride		
Thiothixene		
Tizanidine hydrochloride		
Trifluoperazine hydrochloride		

[a] To calculate the Anticholintergic Risk Scale score for a patient, identify medications the patient is taking and add the total points for each medication.

Reprinted from Rudolph JL, Salow MJ, Angelini MC, McGlinchey RE. The anticholinergic risk scale and anticholinergic adverse effects in older persons. Arch Intern Med 2008;168(5):508–513; with permission.

SUMMARY

The reduction in polypharmacy and avoidance of inappropriate medications is a common goal in the care of older persons, regardless of setting. While multidisciplinary teams and regular medication reconciliation and review can identify and reduce medication-related problems, tools to decrease the use of high-risk/low-benefit medications can help the individual clinician to improve prescribing. Numerous criteria, tools, algorithms, and scoring systems have been developed for use in a wide range of areas from long-term care to the outpatient setting, and some may not be applicable to individual situations. Not all medication review instruments have been adequately validated, and the tools we have presented have varying levels of evidence to support their use. Clinicians also need to be aware of regulatory, policy, and guideline issues that may impact the use of certain criteria for optimum prescribing. Ultimately, optimizing prescribing by reducing polypharmacy and avoiding inappropriate medications is a highly individualized process for each patient, and clinicians will have to use extensive clinical judgment in using the tools presented here.

REFERENCES

1. Weiner BJ, Alexander JA, Shortell SM, et al. Quality improvement implementation and hospital performance on quality indicators. Health Serv Res 2006;41(2):307–34.
2. Reason B, Terner M, Moses McKeag A, et al. The impact of polypharmacy on the health of Canadian seniors. Family Pract 2012. [Epub ahead of print].
3. Richardson K, Ananou A, Lafortune L, et al. Variation over time in the association between polypharmacy and mortality in the older population. Drugs Aging 2011;28(7): 547–60.
4. Qato DM, Alexander GC, Conti RM, et al. Use of prescription and over-the-counter medications and dietary supplements among older adults in the United States. Jama 2008;300(24):2867–78.
5. Routledge PA, O'Mahony MS, Woodhouse KW. Adverse drug reactions in elderly patients. Br J Clin Pharmacol 2004;57(2):121–6.
6. Marcum ZA, Amuan ME, Hanlon JT, et al. Prevalence of unplanned hospitalizations caused by adverse drug reactions in older veterans. J Am Geriatr Soc 2012;60(1):34–41.
7. Loganathan M, Singh S, Franklin BD, et al. Interventions to optimise prescribing in care homes: systematic review. Age Ageing 2011;40(2):150–62.
8. Marcum ZA, Handler SM, Wright R, et al. Interventions to improve suboptimal prescribing in nursing homes: A narrative review. Am J Geriatr Pharmacother 2010; 8(3):183–200.
9. Kaur S, Mitchell G, Vitetta L, et al. Interventions that can reduce inappropriate prescribing in the elderly: a systematic review. Drugs Aging 2009;26(12):1013–28.
10. Beers MH, Ouslander JG, Rollingher I, et al. Explicit criteria for determining inappropriate medication use in nursing home residents. UCLA Division of Geriatric Medicine. Arch Intern Med 1991;151(9):1825–32.
11. Beers MH. Explicit criteria for determining potentially inappropriate medication use by the elderly. An update. Arch Intern Med 1997;157(14):1531–6.
12. Fick DM, Cooper JW, Wade WE, et al. Updating the Beers criteria for potentially inappropriate medication use in older adults: results of a US consensus panel of experts. Arch Intern Med 2003;163(22):2716–24.
13. Aparasu RR, Mort JR. Inappropriate prescribing for the elderly: beers criteria-based review. Ann Pharmacother 2000;34(3):338–46.
14. Budnitz DS, Shehab N, Kegler SR, et al. Medication use leading to emergency department visits for adverse drug events in older adults. Ann Intern Med 2007; 147(11):755–65.
15. Boulkedid R, Abdoul H, Loustau M, et al. Using and reporting the Delphi method for selecting healthcare quality indicators: a systematic review. PLoS One 2011;6(6):e20476.
16. Naugler CT, Brymer C, Stolee P, et al. Development and validation of an improving prescribing in the elderly tool. Can J Clin Pharmacol 2000;7(2):103–7.
17. McLeod PJ, Huang AR, Tamblyn RM, et al. Defining inappropriate practices in prescribing for elderly people: a national consensus panel. Can Med Assoc J 1997; 156:385–91.

18. Barry PJ, O'Keefe N, O'Connor KA, et al. Inappropriate prescribing in the elderly: a comparison of the Beers criteria and the improved prescribing in the elderly tool (IPET) in acutely ill elderly hospitalized patients. J Clin Pharm Ther 2006;31(6):617–26.

19. O'Mahony D, Gallagher PF. Inappropriate prescribing in the older population: need for new criteria. Age Ageing 2008;37(2):138–41.

20. Barry PJ, Gallagher P, Ryan C, et al. START (screening tool to alert doctors to the right treatment)—an evidence-based screening tool to detect prescribing omissions in elderly patients. Age Ageing 2007;36(6):632–8.

21. Gallagher P, Ryan C, Byrne S, et al. STOPP (Screening Tool of Older Person's Prescriptions) and START (Screening Tool to Alert doctors to Right Treatment). Consensus validation. Int J Clin Pharmacol Ther 2008;46(2):72–83.

22. Gallagher P, Baeyens JP, Topinkova E, et al. Inter-rater reliability of STOPP (Screening Tool of Older Persons' Prescriptions) and START (Screening Tool to Alert doctors to Right Treatment) criteria amongst physicians in six European countries. Age Ageing 2009;38(5):603–6.

23. Gallagher PF, O'Connor MN, O'Mahony D. Prevention of potentially inappropriate prescribing for elderly patients: a randomized controlled trial using STOPP/START criteria. Clin Pharmacol Ther 2011;89(6):845–54.

24. Gallagher P, O'Mahony D. STOPP (Screening Tool of Older Persons' potentially inappropriate Prescriptions): application to acutely ill elderly patients and comparison with Beers' criteria. Age Ageing 2008;37(6):673–9.

25. Hanlon JT, Schmader KE, Samsa GP, et al. A method for assessing drug therapy appropriateness. J Clin Epidemiol 1992;45(10):1045–51.

26. Samsa GP, Hanlon JT, Schmader KE, et al. A summated score for the medication appropriateness index: development and assessment of clinimetric properties including content validity. J Clin Epidemiol 1994;47(8):891–6.

27. Hajjar ER, Hanlon JT, Sloane RJ, et al. Unnecessary drug use in frail older people at hospital discharge. J Am Geriatr Soc 2005;53(9):1518–23.

28. Schmader KE, Hanlon JT, Landsman PB, et al. Inappropriate prescribing and health outcomes in elderly veteran outpatients. Ann Pharmacother 1997;31(5):529–33.

29. Wehling M. Multimorbidity and polypharmacy: how to reduce the harmful drug load and yet add needed drugs in the elderly? Proposal of a new drug classification: fit for the aged. J Am Geriatr Soc 2009;57(3):560–1.

30. Frohnhofen H, Michalek C, Wehling M. Assessment of drug treatment in geriatrics with the new FORTA criteria. Dtsch Med Wochenschr 2011;136(27):1417–21.

31. Haque R. ARMOR: a tool to evaluate polypharmacy in elderly persons. Annals of Long-Term Care 2009;17(6):26–30. Available at: http://www.annalsoflongtermcare.com/content/armor-a-tool-evaluate-polypharmacy-elderly-persons. Accessed January 28, 2012.

32. Garfinkel D, Zur-Gil S, Ben-Israel J. The war against polypharmacy: a new cost-effective geriatric-palliative approach for improving drug therapy in disabled elderly people. Isr Med Assoc J 2007;9(6):430–4.

33. Garfinkel D, Mangin D. Feasibility study of a systematic approach for discontinuation of multiple medications in older adults: addressing polypharmacy. Arch Intern Med 2010;170(18):1648–54.

34. Olsson IN, Curman B, Engfeldt P. Patient focused drug surveillance of elderly patients in nursing homes. Pharmacoepidemiol Drug Saf 2010;19(2):150–7.

35. Lapane KL, Hughes CM, Daiello LA, et al. Effect of a pharmacist-led multicomponent intervention focusing on the medication monitoring phase to prevent potential adverse drug events in nursing homes. J Am Geriatr Soc 2011;59(7):1238–45.

36. Drenth-van Maanen AC, van Marum RJ, Knol W, et al. Prescribing optimization method for improving prescribing in elderly patients receiving polypharmacy: results of application to case histories by general practitioners. Drugs Aging 2009;26(8):687–701.
37. Rudolph JL, Salow MJ, Angelini MC, et al. The anticholinergic risk scale and anticholinergic adverse effects in older persons. Arch Intern Med 2008;168(5):508–13.
38. Lowry E, Woodman RJ, Soiza RL, et al. Associations between the anticholinergic risk scale score and physical function: potential implications for adverse outcomes in older hospitalized patients. J Am Med Dir Assoc 2011;12(8):565–72.
39. Kumpula EK, Bell JS, Soini H, et al. Anticholinergic drug use and mortality among residents of long-term care facilities: a prospective cohort study. J Clin Pharmacol. 2011;51(2):256–63.
40. Hilmer SN, Mager DE, Simonsick EM, et al. A drug burden index to define the functional burden of medications in older people. Arch Intern Med 2007;167(8): 781–7.
41. Hilmer SN, Mager DE, Simonsick EM, et al. Drug burden index score and functional decline in older people. Am J Med 2009;122(12):1142–9 e1141–1142.
42. Gnjidic D, Cumming RG, Le Couteur DG, et al. Drug Burden Index and physical function in older Australian men. Br J Clin Pharmacol 2009;68(1):97–105.
43. Lowry E, Woodman RJ, Soiza RL, et al. Drug Burden Index, physical function, and adverse outcomes in older hospitalized patients. J Clin Pharmacol 2011. [Epub ahead of print].
44. Wilson NM, Hilmer SN, March LM, et al. Associations between drug burden index and falls in older people in residential aged care. J Am Geriatr Soc 2011;59(5):875–80.
45. Wilson NM, Hilmer SN, March LM, et al. Associations between drug burden index and physical function in older people in residential aged care facilities. Age Ageing 2010;39(4):503–7.
46. Holt S, Schmiedl S, Thurmann PA. Potentially inappropriate medications in the elderly: the PRISCUS list. Dtsch Arztebl Int 2010;107(31–32):543–51.

Index

Note: Page numbers of article titles are in **boldface** type.

Clin Geriatr Med 28 (2012) 343–348
doi:10.1016/S0749-0690(12)00037-7
0749-0690/12/$ – see front matter © 2012 Elsevier Inc. All rights reserved.

geriatric.theclinics.com

Moving?

Make sure your subscription moves with you!

To notify us of your new address, find your **Clinics Account Number** (located on your mailing label above your name), and contact customer service at:

Email: journalscustomerservice-usa@elsevier.com

800-654-2452 (subscribers in the U.S. & Canada)
314-447-8871 (subscribers outside of the U.S. & Canada)

Fax number: 314-447-8029

Elsevier Health Sciences Division
Subscription Customer Service
3251 Riverport Lane
Maryland Heights, MO 63043

*To ensure uninterrupted delivery of your subscription, please notify us at least 4 weeks in advance of move.

Edwards Brothers Malloy
Ann Arbor MI. USA
May 1, 2012